Secrets of

Sexual

Ecstasy

Carlo de Paoli is a qualified osteopath, practitioner of Chinese Medicine and aromatherapist. He is the ex-principal of the Andrew Still College of Osteopathy and the ex-Chairman of the British and European Osteopathic Association. He is also the founder of the Institute of Traditional Aromatherapy. During the late 'sixties and early 'seventies he lived in the East, for the most part in India, travelling and studying Oriental religion and thought. He speaks many languages and has travelled widely both studying and lecturing. His articles appear regularly in magazines.

Secrets of Sexual Ecstasy

PATHWAYS TO EROTIC PLEASURE

Carlo De Paoli

Marlowe & Company

First published by Bloomsbury Publishing Plc, 1996

This edition published by Marlowe & Company, 1997

Published by
Marlowe & Company
632 Broadway, Seventh Floor
New York, NY 10012

Manufactured in Great Britain

Library of Congress Catalog Card Number: 96-75834

ISBN 1-56924-768-4

Designed by Liz Rowe
Typeset by Hewer Text Composition Services, Edinburgh
Printed by Butler and Tanner Ltd, Frome and London

Secrets of Sexual Ecstasy

CONTENTS

CONTENTS

Love and eros today

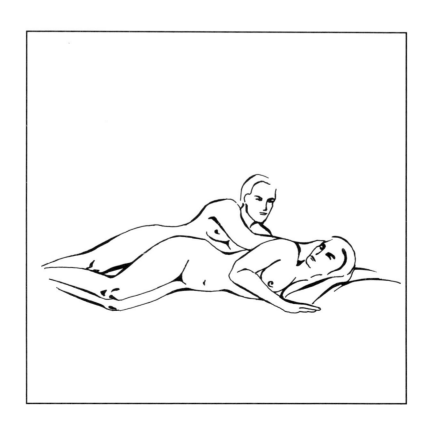

Love Today

U NTIL RECENTLY RELATIONSHIPS seemed easier than today. Most couples met whilst young and learned to cope with their difficulties in relating with a sense of acceptance and sometimes even resignation. Their philosophy was that even if they were to discover soon after marriage that they were not compatible in many critical ways, they could learn how to live with each other for the rest of their lives. The prevailing belief was that people could learn how to love and respect each other with time. And if they failed the message was that they should remain together for the sake of their children and society.

This approach had its advantages: eliminating uncertainty, promoting commitment and encouraging partners to discover profound and tolerant paths to make their union last. Unfortunately this was not always the case and many marriages became loveless and cold, punctuated with either repressed or over expressed anger and frustration. In this sort of family atmosphere children often grew up deprived of affection and warmth to become adults who in turn did not know how to express love and intimacy.

Since the 1960s there has been a radical change of attitudes and consciousness particularly in the Western world. The young have refused to follow in the footsteps of their elders and reconsidered the role of couples and marriages. The new generations have grown up to believe that marriage does not have to be based on a sense of self-sacrifice and denial or on duty and social conformity. On the contrary they believe the union of two people should be based on a sense of individual independence and equality. At the same time couples have become acutely aware of their incompatibilities and are expressing them or feeling them more clearly. This attitude has brought some very important changes in the way marriages and relationships work.

On a positive note partners are encouraged to remain together bound by bonds of mutual understanding and compatibility thus eliminating many forms of social and moral hypocrisy. Few partnerships are now formed out of racial, financial or family considerations, instead they are formed out of love, respect and attraction. On a negative note the vast majority of people caught up in social change were neither emotionally nor mentally prepared for the results. It was as if they had been suddenly catapulted on to totally new territory without any bearings or adequate experience to face this new challenge. We all know that many couples, married and unmarried, now break up as soon as the first signs of difficulty begin to emerge in their relationship. Many people are unable or unwilling to confront the uneasy feelings and fears triggered by emotional problems.

The message of this book is:
- Do not give up so easily!
- Open new paths of relating and new ways to surmount obstacles!

The techniques to achieve these aims are great fun! By presenting new possibilities of touch, eroticism and sexuality I encourage people to open new horizons for their relationships, based on tenderness, joy and both physical and mental communication. This can be a very solid base on which to base a rapport infused with emotional happiness.

Eros

*T*HIS BOOK CONTAINS many sensual and sexual techniques. However, they are not intended to be just a collection of technical or gymnastic skills which could easily become repetitive and mechanical. All these positions and practices are pathways to fulfilled and happy relationships, and all have a spiritual element.

So that you can fully appreciate the meaning of this statement I would like to introduce you to what I mean by *Eros* and *eroticism*. My use of these terms is not the same as their common, modern use; on the contrary I draw on ancient civilisations and ancient ideas, such as Greek and Roman, when I use the terms *Eros* & *eroticism*.

I see *Eros* as the force and inspiration in us which enables us to feel love for life and creation. It makes us appreciate such aspects as touch, colour, melody and aesthetic beauty. It makes us feel alive and glow with excitement. Relationships, particularly in their initial stages, trigger this force in us; this is why we are filled with passion and joy. *Eros* is the god of love, but not only sexual or romantic love. *Eros* is the god of love that extends to all of creation. This is why when we are actually in love we become so appreciative of and grateful for all that life offers us.

Eros is passion for life, the inspiration of the artist, the colour of the painter, the melody of the musician and the muse of the poet.

Sex is a very important part of Eros, but only a part. It follows that a sexual act performed in a skilful way, but devoid of love and tenderness, can leave the participants feeling quite lifeless and empty. So a sexually active person might not be a very erotic person. On the other hand an erotic person might not have, at all times, a sexually active life.

It is worth stressing that most traditional and modern schools of sexuality, both in the East and in the West, have emphasised quality of loving rather than the mere pursuit of sexual conquests or the achievement of constant new positions and techniques.

In this book, *Sexual Healing*, I will assist you in further opening your heart to your lover and to life; you cannot love one person without loving the whole of creation. I will explore with you ways of appreciating fully the beauty and pleasure of touch tenderness, colour and music. We will explore together the most harmonious and healing manifestations of life. It is this love and appreciation of life that we should bring into our relationships as an offering of love. In this way the eroticism shared by the couple can truly become a healing act.

EROS AND YOUR LIFE

The poets say that without the blessings of Eros a lover does not feel excited at the prospect of meeting the beloved, a painter is not attracted to the canvas, a musician neglects his instrument and relationships wither away in dullness and empty silences.

Recognising *Eros* does not mean being filled with a delusive form of excitement which is a denial of how we are really feeling. But even so, it needs to be stressed that in order to lead a full life blessed with happy relationships we need to be open to the colour and vibrancy around us and within us.

Let us conduct a brief check on the level of Eros present in our life:

◆ Look back at those moments in your life, including your childhood, when you truly felt happy and excited about experiencing or witnessing creative and life-enhancing events. Do you still get feelings like that or has the enthusiasm and buoyancy almost disappeared from your life?

- Do you still feel moved and touched by beautiful melodies, colours in the sky, paintings and other aesthetic and artistic manifestations? Or do most things leave you feeling cold and disinterested?
- Are you happy when other people have cause to rejoice or do you feel unhappy and resentful, preferring perhaps to gloat over other people's unhappiness?

If you feel that your life is grey and dull it is time that you made a commitment to yourself to change and uplift your mood. If you are living in such a depressed mood your relationship cannot be a bundle of fun! This book is filled with ways to enhance the quality of your life and relationship and as you read it I am sure you will find plenty of inspiring suggestions to help you change your life for the better.

The most important step

THE MOST IMPORTANT STEP to improve the quality of your life and relationship is to realise that happiness is not purely dependent on external circumstances. On the contrary, you can choose to be happy. If you spend all your life blaming circumstances and the world, nothing will change for the better because external circumstances are always in flux and people might not always behave in a way to make you happy.

You have within the power to see an opportunity for inner growth and development in most circumstances.

When confronted with difficulties many people have a tendency to face them with a pessimistic and negative mind. They focus on the difficult and unpleasant aspects of the situation and fill their minds and hearts with sombre and forbidding visions.

This tendency can strongly affect your relationship in so far as you tend to pay too much attention to the difficult aspects of the liaison and taint joyous feelings towards your lover with depressive moods. We paint the relationship in greys and browns, rather than more vibrant, or subtle colours.

The following visualisation aims to swell your heart and mind with radiant colours and an expansive vision that represents a sense of space and peace. The visualisation will fill you with hope and joy. Of course, life will always present difficult and painful moments but if you can meet them with a positive and loving outlook even the most trying challenges can become a further opportunity for you to become a better human being.

A VISUALISATION TO BRING COLOUR IN YOUR LIFE

Wearing loose clothes, sit or lie comfortably and relaxed. Make sure the room is warm. Dim the lights if you prefer and perhaps burn some incense. In your mind's eye, visualise a large valley covered in a luscious and fertile green mantle. See in it the variety of trees, flowers, streams and birdlife that you really like. Take a deep breath, release it slowly, and give all your attention to your mental picture.

You can hear the carefree and happy singing of birds. Imagine a bright rainbow, on the horizon, quite small.

Now take another deep breath and then release it slowly. See the rainbow slowly grow, filling the entire sky with its radiant colours. Immerse yourself in its beauty for a few minutes.

When you are ready, take another deep breath and release it slowly and say to yourself: 'May my life be filled with the colours of this rainbow'.

Try to practise this visualisation for a few minutes, if not every day, then at least three times a week. After you have finished remain for a few minutes in silence experiencing the feeling generated by this meditation.

You might not begin to harvest its positive results immediately but with time you will not fail to feel better about yourself, your life and your relationship.

Creating and supporting love

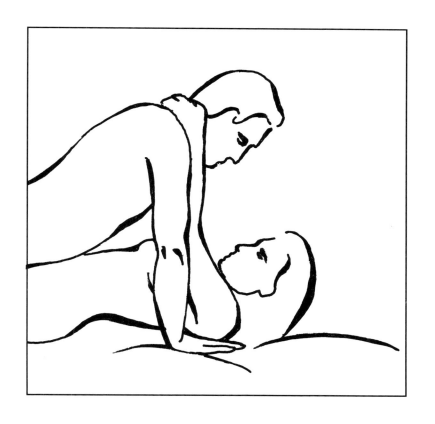

Joyful Sex, Happy Relationships

*I*N THE LAST few years sexologists have shown us various ways to improve our sex lives and I believe that on the whole they have helped. However, from time to time we need to be reminded that the true joy of our love lives is the quality of our relationships.

SEX BORN OUT OF CONFLICT

Some people enjoy sex with a person with whom they have a lot of conflict. Mentally and emotionally antagonism becomes a magnetic pull. However, in both the short and long term, physical attraction born out of friction can wear you out, leaving you emotionally and spiritually starved and empty. Examples of this sort of sexual attraction are when you are physically aroused by:

- a person who is abusive towards you;
- someone who is totally dependent on you;
- someone with whom you never agree on anything but with whom you spend most of your time arguing and fighting;
- anger.

Although these erotic pulls can be very enticing at times, they will leave you hankering for the comfort of true friendship, understanding and support that only a warm and caring relationship can truly offer.

SEX BORN OUT OF LOVE

Although after some time in a relationship sex might not seem as exciting as at the beginning, if you learn to transform it into an act of true sympathy, caring and love it will always bestow on you a great deal of joy.

At the beginning you feel infatuation and a tremendous amount of impetuous attraction and desire. Once the infatuation recedes the physical attraction can also lessen. The aim of this book is to show that the time after the initial infatuation has passed is when you can appreciate a sexuality born out of love and commitment.

I am not talking about a romantic or particularly esoteric concept of love. The love I am talking about is a feeling between two people who have a shared history which enables them to form a bond of friendship and mutual support and whose actions towards each other aim to bring healing and happiness to the relationship.

At this level anxiety about sexual performance lessens and what takes its place is a desire to enjoy each other's company and to give pleasure to one another. This form of sexuality is subtle and gentle but it will keep on growing with time as the relationship deepens in value.

Verbal Communication

*A*T THE BEGINNING of a relationship partners usually find it easy to talk. They say things like, 'We can't stop talking about everything, we share so many things and we have so many dreams in common'. They both want to learn about each other and to share experiences and ideas.

As time goes by this excitement can sometimes start to wane and exciting talk can be replaced by bored conversation, with very few words exchanged. Often one partner reacts to this lack of mental rapport by withdrawing and becoming silent whilst the other becomes even more talkative and frustrated, even ending up being labelled the nagging partner. At the same time many activities that the couple once enjoyed sharing also begin to disappear.

In this state of affairs it is difficult for a joyful sexuality to thrive because, as I have already mentioned, eroticism is at its best when it is born out of full mental and emotional compatibility.

TALK TO EACH OTHER

Whether or not you find it easy to express yourself, it is essential you try to remember the importance of sharing thoughts and feelings with your partner. This means expressing yourself but also allowing and encouraging your partner to do the same. There is nothing worse than someone who talks about themselves incessantly and never stops to ask other people about their interests, ideas, thoughts and feelings.

Whenever you meet with your lover always try to spend

some time talking. Express your feelings, frustrations, dreams and aspirations and let your partner do the same. Ask your partner questions, thus encouraging him or her to delve a bit deeper into themselves. At the end of the conversation you will both feel lighter and happier; your bond will grow stronger because you will see in each other caring friends, not just sexual partners. Any form of eroticism born out of a strong and caring bond will be a truly healing and regenerating experience which will crown and deepen your love.

Blossoming

THIS SECTION HIGHLIGHTS the importance of each individual bringing the best of themselves into the relationship. This might be difficult if you are feeling tense, stressed and unable to find ways to unwind and enjoy the present moment with your partner.

A relaxed and positive person will have much more creativity and joy to bring into the relationship than a person who is tense and frustrated. Tension will knot your muscles, restrict your breathing and clutter your mind with unpleasant thoughts. I am not trying to deny that life can be filled with problems that can make you feel unhappy and tight. But I want to point out that if you view those same problems with a calmer mind you might find it easier to cope with and solve your difficulties.

It is also very important to remember that if you are in harmony with your partner, his or her support will double your strength and capacity, whilst if you tend to dump your frustrations on your partner, you are not only spoiling the relationship but are also weakening yourself.

I have used the word *blossoming* in this context because it means the unfolding or blossoming of the Self through relaxation and positive visualisation. At the same time it means the end of your using the relationship as a depository of your frustrations and tensions. Next I am going to examine various ways in which stress can take hold, and then you can experiment with techniques to halt this unnecessary and harmful build-up of draining energy.

Of course some amount of tension is essential for survival; physically your muscles will collapse without some degree of contraction; mentally you need some aggression and tension to achieve your goals. But if you become unable to let go of tension, you will gradually start living in an unhealthy state of stress, losing your ability to relax, sleep properly, attain serenity or enjoy your life and relationship.

Even if you do not suffer from unhealthy tension now, the following advice will be of great help if you are to avoid its future build-up. By lowering tension levels, not only will you be improving your own well-being, but also your partner's well-being and the happiness of your relationship.

THE LEVELS OF TENSION

There is, of course, an intimate connection between physical, emotional and mental aspects of our being. These three aspects are each, in part, modulated via the nervous system and levels of tension are regulated via the nervous system. I consider tension as existing at four levels; the first two are purely physical, levels 3 and 4 involve the emotions and our mental faculties.

Level 1: Muscular tension

The first level affects the most exterior system, which is the muscular system. Muscles become tense and stiff, particularly around the shoulders, neck and face. This can often lead to symptoms such as recurring tension headaches, uncomfortable muscular soreness in the neck and poor sleep because of an aching body. Tension can then reach other parts, for instance the legs, contributing to conditions such as cramp.

Internal organs, for example the stomach and intestines, are made of a form of muscle and they too can suffer the negative effects of nervous tension, developing such conditions as ulcers or a spastic colon.

Level 2: Respiratory tension

The second level of tension affects the respiratory system. The act of breathing is initiated by muscles controlled by the brain stem and other nerves, such as the vagus. If the normal movement and rhythm of the lungs is disturbed by tension, it can lead to breathlessness or hyperventilation.

Level 3: Emotional tension

If your emotions are affected by tension, you can become panicked, anxious, frustrated or apprehensive even when the situation does not warrant it. You tend to let your imagination run away and to exaggerate things of small significance into major events. When one or both of the partners exaggerates the meaning of most situations and over-dramatises them, the relationship deteriorates because it is conducted in a realm of fantasy, not reality.

Level 4: Mental tension

Finally you reach the mental level when your thoughts start to be distorted by tension. If this happens, your optimism and positivity weaken and you view and judge everything with suspicion and anxiety. Most thoughts become loaded with difficulties, conflicts and disappointments.

Overcoming tension: the art of relaxation

Relaxation exercises can greatly improve your own life and the quality of your relationships. They lower all levels of tension so improve your health, make you more optimistic and positive, help you to view situations in a more balanced context and make you more tolerant and caring. If your musculature and mind are relaxed you can more easily open yourself to the pleasure of touch and sex with your partner.

We shall now practise some relaxation techniques that can de-stress our beings at various levels by decontracting the muscles, freeing the breath, calming the emotions and endowing our thoughts with creativity and positivity.

Sit or lie so that you are comfortable. If you are sitting neither tense your shoulders nor slouch too much; you could place a cushion against your lower back to favour an upright but relaxed position. Make sure that the room is not too stuffy and neither too hot nor too cold. You could play some soothing music, light an incense stick or dim the lighting to create the right mood.

Relaxing your body

Feel the tone of your body musculature. Become aware of the various muscular areas of your body starting from your feet and moving up all the way to your head. Is each muscle group tense or relaxed? At this stage do not try to decontract your muscles, just become aware of their condition. Take note of areas of tension. This will take two to five minutes. Next repeat the same procedure but this time start to relax your muscles. Concentrate your attention on your feet and work your way up to your head. Pass through your calves, knees, thighs, pelvis, buttocks, abdomen, back, neck, face and skull. As you do this, whenever required, will your muscles to relax and decontract. If one muscle group is particularly tense, deliberately tense those muscles even further, take a deep breath, hold for a few seconds and then, whilst breathing out, relax your muscles and feel them decontract.

You can assist the relaxation process by repeating to yourself words or phrases such as, 'Relax', 'I am calm and relaxed', and so forth. You can repeat this procedure a few times, going from your toes to your head and down again. This exercise can last between ten and fifteen minutes at first, but as you become more experienced you might find that you can achieve a state of physical relaxation in a much shorter time.

Relaxing your breath

In this exercise visualise yourself lying in beautiful and calming surroundings. A warm beach with a calm blue sea and clear skies above is an image that most people find calming.

Imagine yourself lying on warm sand. Feel its warmth first on your skin and then let it penetrate and soothe your body.

Enjoy the warmth of the sun and sand, the calmness of the sea and the blue space of the sky.

Now concentrate on the rhythmic and harmonious sounds of waves gently breaking on the beach. Feel your breath entering and leaving your body in a similarly rhythmic and harmonious manner, slow, deep and gentle.

Your body is now soothed and entirely relaxed and your breath is flowing free and deep.

Relaxing your emotions

Now that your body and breath are calm and relaxed you are ready to open your heart centre and expand your capability for unconditional love.

Still visualise yourself lying cosy and relaxed on this beach; your body is comfortable and warm, your breath even and gentle and your mind peaceful and at rest.

Next feel a warm and loving feeling entering your chest. Be grateful and appreciative of being in such a beautiful and comforting place, again concentrate on the sounds of the waves, the chirping of the birds and the warmth of the sun. Extend this sense of love and appreciation to all those people who are close to you and part of your life. Send to each of them this love and as you do so feel it growing stronger and wider. Feel that this love has no boundaries and it fulfils itself just by its capability to give unconditionally.

Offer this love to the whole world, to all the people irrespective of colour, creed or race. Proceed by offering the same to the universe and to all forms of life, including plants and animals.

Once you have completed this visualisation, breathe a bit deeper a few times, stretch your body and gradually bring back your awareness of your surroundings, making a resolution to incarnate in your daily life this state of love and relaxation.

Relaxing your mind

Now let us soothe and relax the mind. Whilst still doing the breathing exercise, feel that you have come to this place for a long period of relaxation and that all your problems have been solved so you are free from all worries. Keep on breathing deeply and freely and enjoy this feeling of ease and comfort.

The warmth of the sun has melted all your worries and the gentle breeze has eased them from your mind.

You now possess the capacity to find a solution to all your problems and troublesome situations by using the strength and calmness of your mind.

By relaxing your mind and releasing your worries with this exercise you might not automatically find a solution to all your problems. However, with a calm mind you will have a better chance of finding your path through life than if you have constantly agitated thoughts and panicked emotions.

At the same time, by releasing tension you will be able to enhance your relationship by facing difficulties and problems in a calm and sensible way.

Once you are quite familiar with all the stages of this meditation you do not need to practise them each time in the given order. For example, sometimes you might feel the need to calm your thoughts in order to move out from a state of confusion. In this case you might practise only two levels, one to calm the breath and one to calm the mind.

At times our lives can be filled with tension and strife and if we do not learn how to deal with it then it becomes easy for these conflicts to enter and sabotage our emotional life and create havoc in our bodies. When we are in a state of tension and inner conflict everything looks gloomy and we become easily irritated and despondent. Every little thing our partner does can make us angry and resentful and we see most things as a personal affront.

These exercises can take us gradually into a different plane of feelings and vision. If we learn the art of relaxation, where we can release destructive feelings and fill ourselves with peace and sympathy, we will be able to look at life and our beloved with a great sense of tolerance and support. If both partners practise these visualisations, their relationship will improve no end.

Recharging: New Vitality

ONCE YOU LEARN how to relax and discharge the four levels of tension that impede your path to a happy and constructive life you are ready to recharge yourself with positive and vibrant energy. You should not underestimate mental exercises based on visualisations as time and again it has been shown how mental concentration can create results on the physical level.

Receiving energy

- Sit comfortably on the floor or on a chair. Keep your back fairly straight but not rigid, with your shoulders and neck relaxed. If you prefer, you can stand, but keep your knees slightly flexed to give you a feeling that your feet are firmly rooted to the ground. Do not arch your back, keep it straight but relaxed.
- Breath deeply, regularly and gently for a couple of minutes to make sure that you are relaxed and alert.
- Lift your arms above your head. Keep the elbows slightly flexed or bent – you do not want to cause muscular tension.
- Turn the palms of your hands towards the ceiling without unduly twisting your wrists. Keep on breathing deeply and gently.
- Visualise a circle of golden energy about one foot above your palms. Feel the warm radiance of this energy, see its halo gently glowing, imagine that it contains peace, vitality and love.
- Next, imagine that this circle of light descends and positions itself on the palms of your hands. Now turn the palms down to face your head and body and visualise that you are pouring this golden light over yourself. Feel it entering your body and penetrating every cell, filling your whole being with radiant and positive energy.
- Now think about your partner and in your mind offer them this positive and healing energy. Say to yourself that you want to be a source of positive thoughts and emotions in the life of the one you love and in the lives of all those you meet.

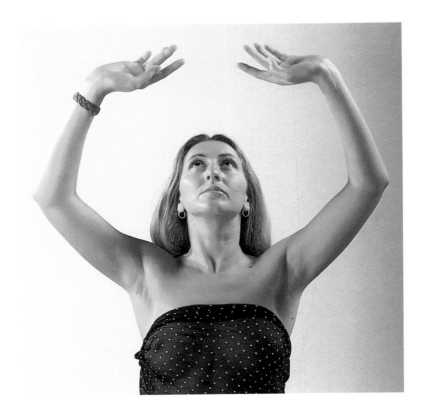

This exercise can help us to become our own dynamo of energy so that besides receiving strength from others we can also become a source of power and inspiration for those we love.

Healing hands

- Sit or stand as in the previous exercise. Shut your eyes, if you prefer. If you are sitting rest your hands on your lap with the palms facing each other at a distance of about 25 cm (10 in).

- Listen to your breath for a couple of minutes until it becomes relaxed and harmonious whilst your body releases any residual tension. Allow your mind to become calm and silent.

- Visualise a small dot of golden light emerging from around your navel area. Your even and regular breath, together with positive and loving thoughts, will allow the golden dot to grow gently and fill your whole abdomen with a pleasant and healing warmth. Concentrate on this warmth for a few minutes.

- Next, feel this golden light and warmth pervade your whole body and being, both mental and emotional, infusing it with vitality and joy. Stay with this feeling for a few minutes.

- Now concentrate on your hands and feel them infuse with this warm and healing golden energy. Stay with this image and feeling for a few minutes.

- Next, imagine yourself touching or massaging someone you love, giving them a sense of joy and well-being.

- With practice you will notice that your hands will become warmer when you do this exercise and people you touch or caress immediately will also notice this effect.

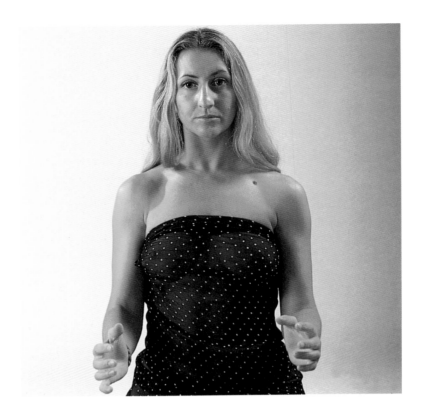

If you practise this exercise daily, your hands will soon develop a permanent healing warmth. Even if you are not aware of this, it will be obvious to those you touch, including your partner.

These two exercises will help you to become a source of positive energy and warmth for yourself and others thus improving your life and the lives of those around you. They are also excellent preparation for sensual massage or love-making.

Touching

WE HAVE ALREADY seen the importance of verbal expression and shall now begin to explore the importance of physical communication. There is not much point in describing sexual positions and techniques if we do not know how to make contact with our skin!

Unfortunately for many men the sexual act consists of achieving an erection and culminating in an orgasm. Our approach encourages a much wider expression of sexuality.

Many people, not just men, believe that metaphorically sex starts and ends in genital orgasm and excitation, but this is not true. All of the body can give great pleasure and every part of the skin is orgasmic in the sense that it can create erotic sensations that are entirely fulfilling. This is why many lovers can sometimes spend hours caressing each other, postponing or even not feeling the need for penetration, totally enjoying the pleasure of touch.

All living beings, not just humans, thrive, grow and survive healthily and happily when there is touch and emotional warmth. Sex without touch and warmth is a cold and mechanical affair that leaves many people frustrated and unfulfilled.

However, for many who are not accustomed to touching or being touched, making this sort of physical contact can be difficult, leaving them feeling odd and embarrassed.

The exercises in this section aim to introduce the beauty of touch and contact and to show how touch can revive and stir all senses and emotions. These exercises are extremely important because they form the basis for all the exercises which follow in later chapters.

Touching an Orange

We are constantly picking up objects, and some of them are very beautiful. But we are so distracted that we tend not to notice what we are holding. In the same way we can touch and be close to our lover without appreciating many of his or her qualities, such as the texture of their skin or their natural fragrance.

This first exercise aims to awaken deep sensations on a daily basis, making you more aware and appreciative of what you can capture with your senses.

- Find a really nice, fresh and bright orange; hold it close to your face with one hand.
- With the other hand gently and slowly caress the orange, using your fingertips. Notice how its skin feels; is it smooth or rugged?
- Take a few deep breaths and inhale its smell. Feed your senses with it.
- Continue to caress the orange and look at it very carefully; appreciate and admire its bright and lively orange colour.
- Thank nature for offering you such a beautiful and delicious fruit.

Touching a Pet

Many people enjoy the presence and company of pets but don't often give them full attention. They ignore the fact that an animal has feelings and the capacity and need to receive and offer a great amount of love.

- Sit next to your pet and, if the animal is receptive, start to stroke it slowly and gently. Feel the silkiness of its skin and fur.

- Feel its subtle reactions when it starts to move and stretch with pleasure. Become aware of which strokes give it the greatest pleasure.

TOUCHING ANOTHER HUMAN

- Sit next to a person dear to you and gently caress him or her. Your touch should be non-sexual. It should convey a feeling of warmth and caring, almost as if it was a parental caress. Perhaps you could concentrate on stroking his or her hair or face, or perhaps a hand or arm – whatever seems appropriate
- The receiver should relax and enjoy the comfort that he or she is receiving.
- It is very important that before we learn how to touch sensually we learn how to touch and caress with a feeling of loving support and tenderness.

TOUCHING YOURSELF

Many people go through life feeling trapped in a body that they neither like nor appreciate. During love-making they can feel blocked and cold because they are ashamed of their bodies so cannot truly receive pleasure. The warm sensations of sensuality are inhibited at skin level and cannot penetrate their muscles. They feel that they are not attractive and do not deserve to be loved.

If you are unhappy with your body, no one can make you feel truly good about it except yourself.

The following exercise can help you achieve this purpose.

- Stand in front of a mirror, preferably naked, and take a good look at your body. Try not to judge, just look at it for a little while, a minute or so.
- Next start caressing yourself with true warmth and

affection. If you start to think that you are not attractive for any reason, imagine that those thoughts are words coming from your body in the mirror.

- Keep on caressing yourself and reassure your body that you love it and that it is as beautiful as it is.
- If you practise this exercise regularly, for a few minutes three times a week, you will notice that your self-caresses become more pleasurable and comforting and that the self-depreciating thoughts from your body will cease.

As you progress through this exercise begin to imagine that your body is telling you: Thanks for your appreciation, I love you too!

In this way you will come to be proud of your looks, at peace with your body and more appreciative of the inherent beauty in everyone.

Sensual Aromatherapy

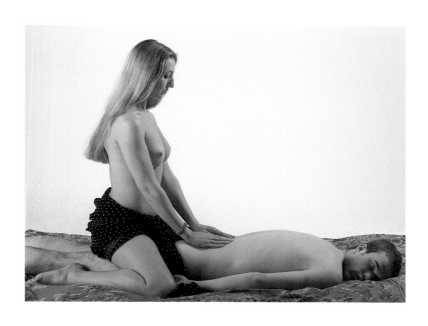

Essential Oils

*P*LANTS, WITH THEIR many parts and components, possess a great amount of life force. When used judiciously they can improve human health and enhance eroticism. In the context of achieving sexual healing their most important role is in sensual aromatherapy.

Many plants contain glands filled with volatile aromatic oil called *essential oil*. This oil gives a plant both a personality, and a unique fragrance. Research shows that one of the main purposes of these oils is defensive. They repel harmful germs and insects that endanger the survival of the plant. For this task they contain many chemicals that are highly antiseptic and so most essential oils have strong anti-bacterial qualities; they preserve tissue and block infections from spreading. The ancient Egyptians were able to preserve mummies indefinitely because they used essential oils, to preserve and protect the body.

Laboratory experiments, conducted particularly in France, have shown that essential oils kill bacteria. This is why they can be used to treat skin infections, grazes and cuts. Some, for instance lavender, have a powerful anti-inflammatory action and are very useful in reducing pain.

Throughout the ages essential oils have been used for cosmetic purposes, either as perfumes or in creams to smooth and strengthen the skin, or in base oils for the purpose of massage. Even today they are the main ingredient of many cosmetic preparations.

Because of their wonderful smells essential oils have been used throughout the ages to enliven and cheer people up. For the same reason they have been used to help promote sexual attraction, as an aid to seduction and to enhance erotic experiences. Many hesitant lovers have given in to their passionate feelings, because they have fallen under the spell of essential oils.

Symbolically, essential oils could be defined as the soul of the plant, denoting a very deep nature. For this reason they can affect humans in a deep manner, awakening many sensations and feelings. Owing to the proximity of the nose to the brain, fragrances reach the central nervous system quickly and rapidly induce various moods. Some researchers now claim that essential oils work on the feeling and sensual areas of our brain – this is why perfumes have always been associated with eroticism and the awakening of sensual emotions.

We all know that sensuality and sex are more than just physical aspects of our being and originate from our emotions and moods. These emotions and moods can favour or inhibit our eroticism. If we are feeling inwardlly repressed and cold our touch will also feel cold and withdrawn. If we are angry and resentful our touch will feel rough and hurtful. Therefore by understanding how different essential oils affect our moods and feelings we can use them to improve our sensual and sexual life.

Methods of use

HERE ARE FIVE primary techniques for employ-
ing essential oils in sensual aromatherapy:

- Before love-making, sprinkle a few drops on your pillow
  or bedding to create an erotic atmosphere and enhance
  your sensual awareness. Alternatively, you could do this
  after love-making to help you fully appreciate the languor
  that follows sexual release.
- Add four or five drops of the chosen oil to your bath. This
  will relax you, and since the fragrance will remain on your
  skin, it will later help you to create an erotic atmosphere.
- Use a diffuser, available from health food shops, to disperse
  the scent of oil in the room where you plan to have sex.
  This will have a captivating and erotically charged effect.
- Use oils as perfume to attract and seduce your partner.
- As part of a sensual massage (see next chapter). When
  blending a personalised massage oil, you will need about
  two soupspoonfuls (thirty to forty millilitres) of base oil for
  every two to three drops of essential oil. When blending
  more than one essential oil, ensure you keep to this ratio.

The choice of essential oil depends not only on their
therapeutic properties, but also on personal taste. You or
your partner may instinctively be drawn to sweet and heady
scents such as jasmine, rose or geranium. On the other hand,
you may prefer the more spicy aromas of rosemary or
peppermint, or the woody scents of cypress or sandalwood. You will need to bear in mind that some people
find strong aromas, such as ylang ylang, sandalwood and
patchouli, overpowering. The best way to find the oil which
appeals to you is to inhale it through the nose for a few
seconds, savouring its aroma and allowing the feeling it

generates to penetrate the body. In this way, you are able to appreciate an essential oil fully, and discover whether it suits you and your partner.

> *Essential oils should never be taken internally. They should also not be used by pregnant women, unless under the supervision of a qualified aromatherapist.*

BLENDING COMBINATIONS

The following aromatic mixtures could help you to create the desired mood either by:

- applying them to your skin;
- adding three or four drops to the bath;
- dropping them on a burner;
- sprinkling them over your sheets.

If you do not want to use the more expensive oils I have added a possible substitute with each formula (in brackets), although if you use just a drop occasionally your expense will be minimal. You can also buy those essential oils diluted in a base oil, even then, their fragrance being so powerful, they retain most of their properties. (Please refer to blending instructions below.)

- To relax, dissipate anger and resentment thus favouring caring and warm sensuality: one drop each of orange peel, chamomile (lavender) and geranium.
- To relax, remove anxiety and tension thus favouring a relaxed and trusting form of sensuality: one drop each of lavender, geranium and neroli (orange peel).
- For individuals who cannot open up to love because of painful past experiences and the fear of being hurt again: two drops of rose (rosewood) and one drop of sandalwood.

- To remove guilt and encourage a sense of pure and uninhibited joyous and spontaneous pleasure: two drops of jasmine and one of ylang-ylang. If you do not want to use jasmine you can mix two drops of ylang-ylang and one drop of either geranium or vetiver.

- For people who tend to feel reserved and are sexually inhibited: mix two drops of rosemary and one of ginger. This mixture will warm them physically, emotionally and spiritually.

- For people who tend to be a bit mechanical in their love-making or lack a sense of fantasy: mix one drop of geranium, one of orange peel and one of ylang-ylang.

The Properties of Some of the Main Essential Oils

MANY ESSENTIAL OILS extracted from plants all over the world are in use today and as aromatherapy becomes more popular more oils are being introduced all the time. In this book I am going to discuss the main properties of a few essences which are frequently used in sensual aromatherapy.

I shall concentrate on sensual aspects of the oils but I would like to remind you once again that each individual is different and essences might act in different ways in different individuals.

Essential oils can be expensive, but you only use a tiny amount at any one time, thus spreading the cost. It is possible to buy ready prepared massage oils and this is an effective, but affordable option.

Chamomile/Camomile

(*Anthemis nobilis*)

These pleasant-looking, small yellow flowers have a marked effect on the nervous and digestive systems, particularly when digestive upsets are caused by stress and worrying. For this purpose chamomile can be massaged over the abdomen. Like lavender, chamomile is also a good analgesic, which means that it can be used whenever pain is present. It is also anti-inflammatory, and therefore useful for irritated and sore skin, and can be recommended for restlessness and insomnia.

Sensual effects

Chamomile helps during love-making when a person feels tense, particularly with a contracted and taut abdomen. Nervous tension and anxiety can often block digestion and contract the abdomen. Chamomile dissolves stomach butterflies and relaxes the lovers in the present moment. It is also reputed to dissipate irritability and resentment that can greatly hinder the expression of our loving sensuality.

Cypress

(*Cupressus sempervirens*)

The essential oil is extracted from the leaves and cones of the tree. It is mainly used on the circulatory system where it exerts a stimulant and astringent action. It strengthens the valves of the veins, helping in conditions such as varicose veins, and it promotes the flow of blood throughout the body. However, remember not to massage over varicose veins; rather apply the oil in distal areas, for instance the feet.

Sensual effects

Cypress is indicated for individuals who tend to get poor circulation not only on a physical plain but also an emotional one. They do not find it very easy to flow with the situation and tend to become inhibited by limbs that are always too cold or too hot.

The coniferous fragrance of cypress makes these individuals more open to move their limbs, particularly their hands, in tune with their inner sensual feelings.

Geranium

(Pelargonium odorantissimum)

The sweet scent of this plant is a favourite of many and it reflects its healing powers. The actions of geranium are balancing and soothing. It is gently calming but it does not sedate, it tonifies without exciting. It will promote relaxation leaving you alert and fresh. It is also an excellent anti-inflammatory, helping skin conditions characterised by redness and dryness.

Sensual effects

Geranium will relax the lovers whilst at the same time enhancing their romanticism and their capacity to transport themselves into a more dreamy and fantasy-like world. It also triggers feelings of 'sweetness' and caring, encouraging the lovers to touch each other with a loving mood rather than in a mechanical and cold manner.

Jasmine

(Jasminum officinale/Jasminum grandiflorum)

If you have smelled the flowers of jasmine during a warm summer's night you will easily understand its actions. It livens the heart, opens the chest and lifts depression. It increases vitality without over-heating the system, unlike some hot essential oils.

Sensual effects

Jasmine encourages joy and enthusiasm. It removes sexual blockages caused by a sense of sin and guilt, restoring a sense of sexual innocence and spontaneity. Once guilt and fear can be emotionally and physically released the body can be opened up to an ocean of sensual ecstasy. Jasmine shows us how to enjoy pleasure without inhibitions.

According to my experience it is the best and safest aphrodisiac, for which purpose it should be massaged over the lower back.

Lavender

(Lavandula vera/Lavandula officinalis)

Lavender is probably one of the most popular essential oils and its applications are many and potent. Its most marked action is on the nervous system where it acts as a sedative useful for anxiety, insomnia and hysteria. It calms pain and is used for various complaints such as neuritis or nerve pain, for instance sciatica or trigeminal neuralgia. Lavender can also be applied over areas of trauma, for instance when there has been a blow on the body. It is anti-irritant and anti-inflammatory and can be used for such varied conditions as irritated skin and bee stings. Lavender also disinfects and helps to heal cuts and abrasions, and improves circulation and muscular cramps. However, it should not be used more than twice a week for a body massage because of its potent sedative qualities.

Sensual effects

Lavender helps people who are excessively shy and tense and who accumulate a tremendous amount of anxiety during an erotic session. Tension can sometimes be so pronounced that on occasions they can feel faint, short of breath and have a cold sweat. The fragrance of lavender will promptly decontract them and make them feel relaxed, revitalised and ready to participate in loving acts with their lover.

Neroli

(Citrus vulgaris)

This oil is extracted from the flowers of the bitter orange from Seville in Spain and is considered one of the best calming and relaxing oils without being too sedative or creating drowsiness. It is recommended for insomnia, anxiety and stress.

Sensual effects

In love-making neroli can relax and soothe, whilst at the same time creating a sense of curiosity and excitement. It is an oil that I often recommend to use in whichever form you choose – in the bath, with a diffuser, on your skin or on the pillow – before love-making to encourage relaxation and enhance sensuality, or afterwards to enjoy further the languor that follows a sexual encounter.

Orange peel
(Citrus aurantium)

A popular natural medicament used throughout the world and extensively used in Chinese medicine. It promotes good digestion and is particularly helpful in relieving constipation, for which purpose you can massage it over the abdomen.

Sensual effects

Many people love the effect of citrusy scents giving them fantasies and feelings of being caressed by a light, fragrant breeze on a warm summer's night. If you would like to create a similar atmosphere during your love-making this is definitely the oil for you!

Peppermint
(Mentha piperita)

This oil acts primarily on the digestive system, stimulating and speeding all the digestive processes. It calms the effects of flatulence, belching and abdominal swelling and has a general stimulant and refreshing effect over the whole body. Peppermint is also widely used to help relieve the symptoms of colds and flu and can be helpful to assist expectoration.

Sensual Effects

If you like the fragrance of this oil, you could use it to stimulate the senses and awaken the mind, particularly if you have had a tiring day, or if you feel a little fuzzy in the head because of a cold or similar complaint. Peppermint will help you to become alert, dynamic and therefore able to participate fully with your partner during love-making.

Rose

(Rosa damascena/Rosa gallica)

It is rare to find someone who is not captivated by the fragrance of roses and their essential oil. Roses are truly the flowers of love! They are an aphrodisiac, not in the sense that they arouse the heat and passion of sex but more in the sense that they relax, create trust and open the heart to love. Roses help to regulate irregular and painful periods and in antiquity they were reputed to increase fertility in women. They are anti-inflammatory and slightly astringent, therefore useful for inflamed, lax and dry skin conditions. They cleanse the liver and help the digestive system particularly when there is heat and inflammation leading to conditions such as ulcers and ulcerative colitis. Rose can cheer up a depressed mind and encourage relaxation, but is not sedative in any way.

Sensual effects

Rose is reputed to help individuals who have been emotionally hurt to the point where they cannot trust their feelings for love and sexuality any more; they are always anxious that the next encounter is going to bring even more pain. Rose opens them up again to the fragrance and beauty of love with a sense of abandonment and trust.

Rosemary

(Rosmarinus officinalis)

Rosemary is a stimulant, tonic and warming essential oil. It promotes circulation to all the body parts and is recommended to strengthen a blood flow to the brain for people with symptoms such as poor memory and concentration. It stimulates the liver, increases the appetite and can be use for cold and lethargic individuals who have a tendency to poor circulation and cold extremities. However, rosemary should be avoided by people with high blood pressure and all other complaints accompanied by a sensation of heat and inflammation.

Sensual effects

Rosemary helps people with low sexual drive who feel cold towards and are easily intimidated by sex. Often these individuals have a very tight and congested chest and upper body, whilst their pelvis and genital area feels cold and numb. Rosemary restores circulation, warmth and drive to the lower part of the trunk and particularly to the genital area.

Sandalwood

(*Santalum album*)

The oil of this wood is widely used in eastern countries, particularly in India, where it is highly regarded as an agent that promotes peace of mind, meditation and spiritual thoughts. For this reason some religious people apply sandalwood paste to their foreheads before they pray or meditate. It encourages clear and peaceful thinking in difficult and conflicting situations. Sandalwood is also widely used for the relief of urinary infections such as cystitis and NSU (non-specific urethritis) probably because of its anti-inflammatory and soothing nature.

Sensual effects

Sandalwood brings a sensation of peace and harmony between the lovers creating a sense of spiritual unity between them. It helps individuals who cannot let go of their confused thoughts, fears and existential conflicts even during lovemaking. Sandalwood 'cools' their heads and helps them to relax with a sense of calmness and peaceful thinking.

Vetiver

(Andropogon muricatus)

Vetiver has a very sweet and deep fragrance and is a popular essence in the East. Vetiver produces a sense of pleasant languor and relaxation whilst at the same time awakening and refreshing the mind. Like rose and jasmine, vetiver has sensual overtones. It is also considered beneficial for circulation, particularly for those who suffer from hot and inflamed extremities.

Sensual effects

Vetiver helps the lovers first to relax and enjoy sensuality and then to awaken and maintain deep overtones of sexual intensity. It also helps lovers to express sexual fantasies and dreams, something many of us are reluctant to do, but which, if done with respect and innocence, can greatly heighten the sexual communion of the couple.

Ylang-Ylang

(Cananga odorata)

The essential oil is extracted from the flowers of a tree which grows particularly in the Philippines, Indonesia and Madagascar. It has a sweet scent and is highly popular in those countries as a relaxant and aphrodisiac.

Sensual effects

Ylang-ylang is prescribed for situations of sexual inadequacy where the cause is anxiety and apprehension. It promotes serenity with a sense of joy. When using this oil just think of the colours, fragrance and joy of the Pacific Islands where sex is regarded as a beautiful and uplifting gift of nature.

Sensual Massage

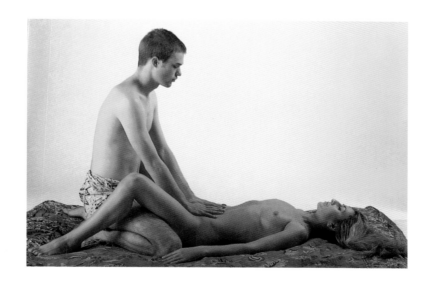

*S*ENSUALITY IS AT THE root of a happy sexual rapport and touch is at the root of sensuality. Massage is a way to expand and structure the limitless possibilities of touch. Many of us fail to realise the beauty and healing power of a massage given with love and care, both at a physical and emotional level.

Massage is as old as human touch. Even animals know its benefits and use many methods to stroke and fondle each other.

Even plants thrive on caring touch. Hundreds of scientific experiments have shown that plants are endowed with a form of intelligence and with feelings. It has been shown that they respond to touch, words and even to thoughts. Plants that are regularly touched and sent loving thoughts grow more strongly than plants that have been deprived of this care. If this is what touch can do for plants, think what it could do for a loving human relationship. If both partners touched each other with warmth and endeavoured to send each other positive and supportive thoughts, the relationship would flourish.

In many historical texts from ancient cultures there are references to the benefits of massage. It is mentioned in cultural and medical texts from China, India, Egypt, Greece, Rome and Arabia. In ancient Egypt massage was taught in temples as a sacred art, alongside herbal medicine and various forms of religious ritual and divination.

Massage was also used in all those cultures, and in particular by the Romans, as a form of relaxation and as a beauty treatment. Base oils were mixed with essential oils and herbs and applied – by various techniques – all over the body to regenerate and beautify the skin, particularly facial skin.

The Benefits of
Sensual Massage

*T*HE BENEFITS OF massage are many and various. Sensual massage has its own particular healing properties. The main ones are as follows:

- It brings couples together at all levels – physical and emotional, mental and spiritual.
- It aids healing – often relationships can become slack and difficult because too much attention is paid to emotional and mental obstacles. Massage and touch cut through those difficulties, bypassing the mind and concentrating the attention of the partners on touch, closeness and healing. Where there is separation it brings closeness, it transforms coldness into warmth, rage into passion and it can bridge gaps no other method can.
- It encourages sexual attraction. After some years together many couples lose sexual attraction towards one another. This could be due to some form of incompatibility, but more often than not the cause is a form of boredom that sets in with repetition, particularly if their earlier sexual rapport was mainly penetrative. Sensual massage is the gate to a more varied and deeper physical rapport which will allow the expression of old feelings. For those couples who have not experienced a weakening in their sexual attraction sensual massage is the gate to further dimensions of erotic pleasure and closeness.
- It removes stress and encourages a rosy outlook on life. It can relieve stress-related disorders, for instance headaches, indigestion and insomnia.
- It encourages physical stamina. Gently squeezing and

stimulating the muscles improves circulation, removes toxic build-up, and eases minor aches, such as back ache. It also stimulates the flow of lymph, which favours the elimination of toxins and strengthens the immune system.

Preparing for Sensual Massage

MAKE SURE THAT the room has been well ventilated so it is not stuffy, but that it is warm enough for the receiver not to feel cold. Dim the lights if you prefer, and perhaps play some soft music or light an incense stick.

Fill a saucer with a good base oil obtained from a health food shop. Sunflower, corn, almond or grape seed are all good oils to use. Add two or three drops of an essential oil. See chapter 00. Just pour enough oil in your hands to lubricate the area you will be working on. Add more as and when necessary.

Do not worry if at first you do not feel confident in your strokes. With time and practice you will become more familiar and versatile with the techniques. I have illustrated an introductory massage sequence. However, with time you will learn to trust your intuition and create your own strokes, most of which will emerge as you are practising.

The main massage term that I use is *effleurage*, derived from the French word *effleurer* which means to touch lightly. Effleurage is basically a long and continuous stroke by the hands using medium to light pressure. It aims to relax and to promote circulation and well-being. In the context of a sensual massage effleurage could almost be translated as 'caressing' because it denotes a gentle and sensual touch that aims to create pleasure and relaxation.

Do not massage over recent scars, lumps or growths. If you suffer from any medical condition consult your doctor prior to receiving a massage. It is best to avoid using essential oils during pregnancy, particularly during the first six months, unless you are under the supervision of, or being treated by, a qualified and experienced aromatherapist.

Sensual Massage: an introductory sequence

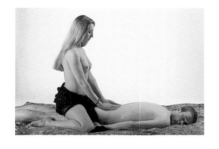

This is a good position for a back massage as it creates a pleasant body contact and allows the giver to reach every part of the back.

- Sit astride your partner, just on the lower part of their buttocks.
- Keep only a light contact: do not put too much weight on them.
- Avoid sitting on their legs because this could be rather uncomfortable for them.

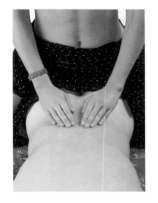

This stroke is a very good way to start a massage session. It relaxes the receiver, creating a sense of trust and sensuality.

- Apply oil to both hands and position them at the base of your partner's spine.
- Breathe in and whilst breathing out glide your hands towards the shoulders, keeping the spine between them.
- Reach the shoulders and follow their contours with gentle but even and steady pressure.
- Slightly relax the pressure and bring your hands down the back to the base of the spine, massaging the sides of the

body with your hands open and fingers pointing outward as you do so.

- It is important to perform this stroke with the whole hand, not just the fingers.
- Return your hands to the base of your partner's spine and repeat the stroke a few more times.

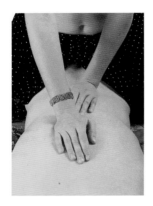

This effleurage stroke revitalises the spine, awakens sensuality and removes tiredness.

- Place one hand on top of the other at the base of your partner's spine and rub the spine in an upward movement, first with one hand and then with the other.
- Start with the hand that is on top and as soon as it reaches the base of the neck return it to the base of the spine and repeat the movement with the other hand.
- The pressure should be light and pleasurable.
- Repeat the stroke for a few minutes and keep an even and regular rhythm.

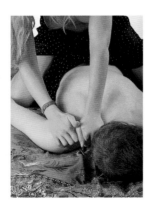

Sexual fears and tension in general accumulate a great deal around the shoulders contributing to problems such as tension headaches and insomnia. This is why many people feel so relieved, sometime ecstatic, when their shoulders are massaged.

- Knead around your partner's right shoulder with both hands in rhythmic fashion starting from the base of the neck and working outward to the tip of the shoulder.
- Knead your way back to the neck and repeat the massage on the left shoulder.
- Practise the stroke for two or three minutes on each shoulder.

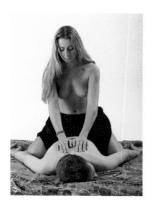

This is similar to the first effleurage technique over the whole back.

- Using the whole of your hand, place both hands either side of your partner's spine on the upper back.
- Repeat the stroke for three or four minutes.
- Move your right hand in a clockwise direction and your left hand in an anticlockwise direction, keeping the movement over the upper shoulders.

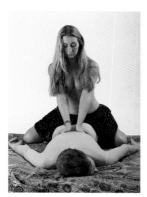

This technique helps to relieve lower back ache and increases circulation in the lower part of the body, thus also increasing vitality around the sexual organs.

- Again, using the whole of your hands, place one on each side of the spine, parallel to the waist-line, and massage the lower back using clockwise and anticlockwise movements.
- Include the buttocks as well.
- Practise the stroke for two or three minutes.

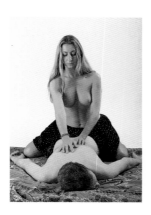

This feathering technique is a very good way to conclude a back massage.

- Using your fingertips, lightly stroke your partner's back first with one hand, then with the other, from the base of their neck to the base of their spine.
- Keep the movement smooth and rhythmic.
- If your partner is ticklish ask them to breathe deeply and slowly while you make firmer contact. With time they will be able to relax more and receive and enjoy this stroke fully.

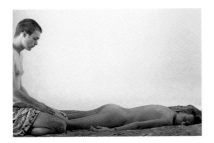

This technique promotes circulation and helps relieve leg cramp and muscular pain as well as transmitting the sensual feelings generated in the back, all the way down to the legs and feet.

- Sit on your heels to one side of your partner's lower legs. Your partner should be lying face down.
- Rest your hands for a few seconds above their ankles to make contact with their body.
- Begin this effleurage by breathing in, then as you breathe out glide your hands with gentle pressure over the middle of their leg all the way to the top.
- Glide your hands back down their leg with fingers pointing outward. This movement should be even and smooth.
- Repeat two to three times on each leg.

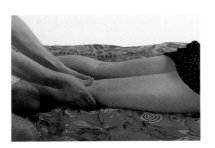

Not many people realise how pleasurable the back of the knee can feel when it is rubbed. This light touch can help you to realise that erotic pleasure can be found everywhere in the body.

- Sit next to your partner, who should be lying face down. With the pad of one thumb and then the other rub gently round the back of your partner's knee covering the whole area.
- Repeat the technique on your partner's other knee.
- Practise the massage for one to two minutes on each knee.

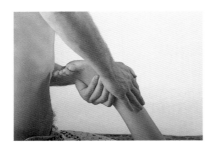

Most people adore having their feet rubbed, bringing solace to a hard day's work or just increasing one's enjoyment and sensual pleasure. Practise it for three or four minutes.

- Sit next to your partner's lower legs. Lift their right lower leg and rest it against your left knee for comfort and stability.
- With both hands cupped hold one side of their ankle.
- Massage the other side of their foot and ankle with a sweeping and gentle effleurage then repeat the stroke on the opposite side of the same foot.

- Perform the same procedure on your partner's other foot.
- Keep a secure and steady hold while using your whole palm to create a pleasurable and warm sensation all over your partner's feet.

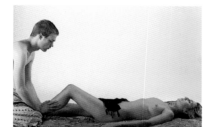

- Ask your partner to lie on their back.
- Bend their leg slightly with her foot resting between your knee and the floor. This will give the leg stability and support.
- Place your hands just above their ankle area.
- Breathe in and as you breathe out glide your hands along the middle of the leg until they reach the top of the thigh.
- Wrap your hands around the thigh and then return to the starting position by gliding your hands down the leg with your fingers pointing outward along each side of the leg.
- Allow the movement to have a smooth and even rhythm.
- Repeat the technique on your partner's other leg.
- Perform the stroke three to four times on each leg.

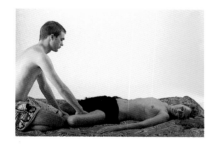

- Keeping the same position as above place your right hand on top of your partner's knee and gently push their leg as far as it will comfortably reach.
- Rest your left hand on the right leg and with your right hand massage the inner right thigh.
- Start by placing your right palm with fingers facing the floor just above the inner knee and sensually rub the inner thigh up to close to the genitals.
- Turn your palm outward and return to the starting position.
- Repeat two to three times, then perform the procedure on your partner's left leg.

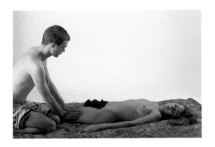

- Sit on your heels to one side of your partner's lower legs.
- Rest your hands for a few seconds above their ankles to make contact with their body.
- Start this effleurage by breathing in and as you breathe out glide your hands with gentle pressure over the middle of the leg all the way to the top.
- Return to the ankle by gliding your hands down the leg, with one hand on each side of the leg with your fingers pointing outward. This movement should be even and smooth.
- Repeat the stroke two to three times.
- Perform the procedure on your partner's other leg.

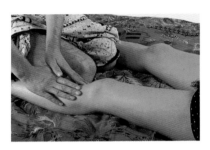

- Place the tips of the fingers of each hand together just beneath the middle of the lower joint of the knee.
- Guide your hands upwards and when you reach the middle of the upper joint rub gently in a circular motion with each hand massaging one side of the knee.
- Repeat the technique two or three times, then perform on your partner's other knee.

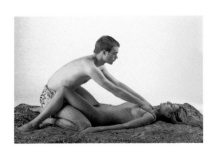

This technique is highly arousing while at the same time improving digestion and respiration.

- Ask your partner to lie on her back while you sit on your heels with your knees comfortably open to the sides.
- Place their legs across your thighs.
- Rest your hands palms down just above the pubic area at the base of the abdomen.
- Hold them in this position for a few seconds to make contact.
- Take a deep breath and start rubbing along the middle of the torso all the way up to the base of the neck.
- Turn your hands to the sides with your fingers pointing outward and glide them down the sides of the body, returning to the original position.
- Repeat five or six times.

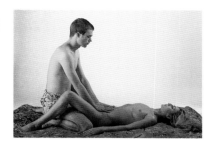

- Remain in the same position. This time place the palms of your hands with fingers pointing outward on the crease where your partner's thighs meet their trunk.
- Massage down the legs rubbing along the outer legs until you reach the knees.
- Return to the original position by massaging the inner thigh with the tips of your fingers pointing towards the floor.
- Repeat five or six times.

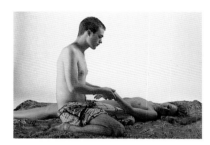

- Take your partner's right arm and hold it by the wrist at an angle of about 45 degrees.
- With your left hand rub the inner part of their arm with a gliding movement.
- Start from the wrist and reach the shoulder with your fingers pointing toward the ceiling.
- Then, turn the hand down and glide your fingers back to the wrist.
- Change hands, hold the wrist with your left hand and massage the outer part of the arm with your right hand.
- Repeat two to three times on each arm.

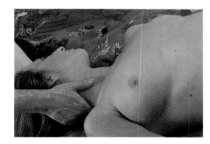

This is a very useful stretch for the neck, an area which can become tense and sore, creating problems such as headaches.

- Slowly turn your partner's neck to the side, resting their head on your left hand.
- With your right hand gently hold the muscle on the side of the neck between your thumb and palm.
- Starting from the area where her neck meets the skull glide your hand all the way down to the shoulder.
- When you reach the shoulder repeat the movement back towards the head.
- Repeat three to four times.
- Perform the technique on the other side of your partner's neck.

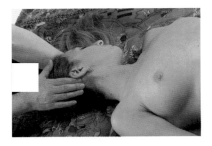

I have yet to meet someone who does not enjoy having the backs of his or her ears caressed. This is a very soothing, pleasurable and sensual technique which can create the right mood for love-making.

- Hold your partner's head as in the previous stroke and caress up and down behind their ear with your fingertips. Repeat it for two to three minutes.
- Repeat the stroke on your partner's other ear.

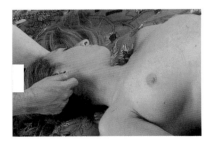

This is also a very pleasurable and sensual massage stroke.

- Hold your partner's head to one side and massage their ear with your thumb and index finger particularly around the lobe area. The movement is gliding and pinching.

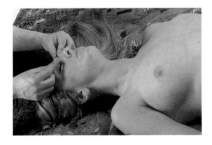

- Sit on the floor behind your partner.
- With your index finger and thumb gently pinch along the whole length of the eyebrow.
- Start from the root of the nose and return to it.
- Repeat two to three times on each eyebrow.

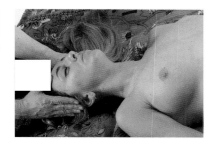

The next two techniques are very good to relax the face and postpone the arrival of wrinkles.

- Place both thumbs together at the top of your partner's forehead, close to the hairline.
- Slowly glide both thumbs with firm but not hard pressure to the sides of the forehead.
- Glide thumbs back to the starting position.
- Repeat this process twice.
- Next repeat the same stroke on the middle part of the forehead, then on the lower part, just above the eyebrows.
- If you wish you can repeat the whole sequence, but this time begin from the bottom part of the forehead.

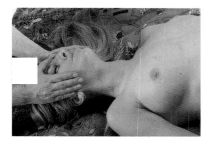

This is a very good stroke to conclude a massage with as it will leave your partner in a state of languid relaxation, drifting off into clouds of delight!

- Wrap your partner's whole face in the palms of your hands and slowly rub upwards towards the temples, slightly pulling the skin towards you. This technique is very good to strengthen sagging face muscles.

The path of ecstasy

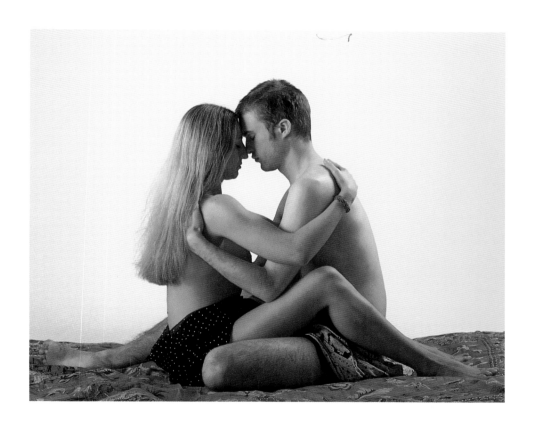

Eastern Philosophy

*B*EFORE I DESCRIBE the history and practice of Tantra and Tao I would like to describe the main difference between Eastern and Western thought because this will help you to place the traditions of India and China in context.

Our religious and spiritual way of looking at life has a clear dualistic tendency. We view the world almost as if it were a corruption of a heavenly idea and many people think we need to seek divine forgiveness in order to reach heaven after death. They believe entry to heaven can be achieved by following a series of commandments while we are in the material world then, after death we will be granted eternal life in the contemplation of Divinity.

According to Eastern thought, particularly the Chinese school of Taoism and the Indian schools of Tantra and Vedanta everything is a manifestation of the same life force or Ch'i. This life force can express itself at various levels of *condensation*, on the mental and spiritual levels it is more rarefied whilst on the material plain it is more solid. Therefore we can say that there is a level of pure existence, the Tao, or according to Hinduism, the Brahman, and gradually this force manifests itself in descending forms of existence – the mind, the emotions, the vital breath and the material body.

Each level is interconnected and a part of the same energy. According to Vedanta, a non-dualistic Indian spiritual school, and Tantrism, the process of enlightenment consists of the individual shedding the illusion that it is separate from the whole and realising its unity with the unborn and eternal spirit. It is only our mind enveloped by the power of illusion that sees duality in everything and life as a struggle between the single parts. When we discard illusion we remember our true nature and the nature of all beings. Then and only then can we live in peace with ourselves and the world.

When we see our unity with the whole of creation we cannot hurt others any more because we feel their pain as our own. Thus individual freedom leads to universal love.

At this level we still exist as individuals but we are free from the pain of duality and are blessed with the presence of spirit.

Tantra tends to emphasise the transcendental aspect of the mystical experience and many of its sexual exercises aim to create a state of spiritual communion. Taoism emphasises the positive aspects of a life led in harmony with nature and Taoist exercises emphasise health-giving properties.

However, both Tantra and Tao are very similar and the sexual positions and meditations are often almost identical.

HEALING PATHWAYS

As I have just said, according to this Eastern approach we not only possess a physical body consisting of flesh and bones but we are also pervaded by subtle currents of energy or Ch'i that sustain our physical life. All of our mental and emotional activities are regulated by psychic centres or *Chakras*. The aim of spiritual practices including the sexual ones is to harmonise these subtle currents, or *meridians*, and chakras. When this is achieved we can experience good health and joyful emotions and couples can become a source of love and healing for each other.

When the One whose original essence is pure existence and bliss becomes the many he expresses different qualities; creativity, joy and power. These in turn become spiritual and mental aspects and propensities of the individual soul – the capacity to have will power, joy, direction and so forth. These qualities create the various elements of creation, such as fire, water, air and earth, each manifesting an aspect of nature, for instance fire becomes joy, water becomes will power, and so on. The elements then create matter and the body. The body is permeated by these subtle creative and vital forces.

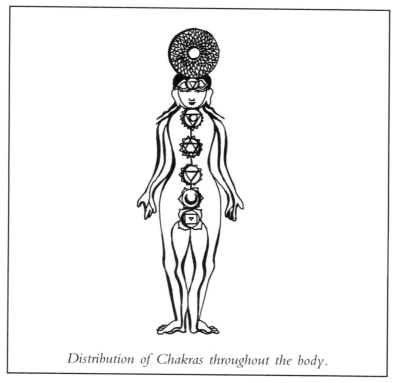

Distribution of Chakras throughout the body.

Taoism sees these forces as flowing through the human body as meridians or energy currents. Tantra shares this vision but places more emphasis on energetic meeting points along the trunk and head, i.e. the chakras.

Each meridian is connected to an organ and meridian and organ influence and regulate each other. For example, a congested gall-bladder could give you a pain in the shoulder where its meridian passes.

The most important aspect to understand about meridians or chakras is that they not only control a body area but also an emotion and spiritual quality of our life. For example, the kidneys are associated with will power, therefore, by tonifying the kidney meridian we can also strengthen the will power of the individual.

The Ultimate Quest

*A*CCORDING TO MOST spiritual schools the soul of the individual constantly yearns to reunite itself with its source and to experience again a state of unity. Unaware of this we humans seek fulfilment in external objects, searching beyond ourselves for something that is really within us. We do not realise that all material forms are in constant flux and change, nothing is permanent. Thus we are often in emotional pain, and it is only when we rediscover our true sources and natures that we can achieve peace. The path of the lovers who practise sexual healing is to become a fountain of inspiration and love for each other and to assist one another in rediscovering their ultimate nature.

THE LEFT- AND RIGHT- HANDED PATHS

Both Chinese and Indian religious words can be translated and interpreted in various ways. I think the best interpretation of *Tantra* is *tool to expand consciousness*. Tantra is more magical in its nature, at least in so far as it uses rituals with gestures (*mudras*), invocations (*mantras*), symbols (*yantras*) and various offerings. There are two Tantric paths, the right-handed and the left-handed.

The right-handed Tantra follows a meditative path and it advocates a life that tends to material and worldly renunciation.

The left-handed Tantra, on the contrary, uses sexuality to achieve a spiritual realisation. Its premise is that in this present material world if we try to suppress our senses we only strengthen them and we risk being overwhelmed by our erotic frustration. Therefore our best strategy is to make friends with our senses, particularly with our sexuality and to use it to transcend our sense of division and duality.

Tao could also be translated in various ways, but my favourite interpretation is *the path of wholeness*. Those Taoist masters who chose to accept sexuality did so in the understanding that a happy sexual life can allow us to follow the path of harmony with nature, thus benefiting our health and promoting a longer life.

Yin and Yang

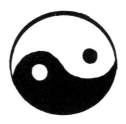

The Yin Yang symbol.

The Tao
gives birth to the One;
The One
gives birth to the two;
The Two
give birth to the three;
The three give birth to every living thing.
All the things are yield in Yin, and carry Yang:
And they are held together in the Ch'i of teeming energy.

IN ORDER TO appreciate fully the path of sexual union we need to understand the concept of polarities in Eastern thought. For the one to manifest creation it needs to become two and life force must have polarity to flow from one to the other. The

Taoists called this duality at the base of all life *Yin* and *Yang*, Hindus call it various names such as *Shiva* and *Shakti* or *Vishnu* and *Lakhsmi*.

The Yin is the more receptive pole; it is night, moon, cool, winter, rest and sleep, earth, shape and form. Yang is the more expansive pole; it is day, sun, hot, summer, activity and expansion, sky, shapeless energy and movement. These two poles are totally interdependent, there could be no night without day, no summer without winter, no expansion without rest. They also contain each other; everything that is Yang has Yin in it and vice versa. The important thing to understand is that although they look like opposite poles they are only the manifestation of the same energy, or as the Chinese call it *Ch'i*. When Ch'i becomes the night it is called yin, when it becomes the day it is called Yang.

The male appearance has a more Yang shape, the female appearance is more Yin, the penis and semen are more Yang whilst the vagina and ovaries are more Yin. However, it would be wrong to classify man as Yang and woman as Yin because a man can have many Yin qualities while a woman can have many Yang qualities. In the sexual act both man and woman can assume either Yin (receptive) or Yang (assertive) roles.

When two lovers come together as one their Yin and Yang poles unite and harmonise and together they can achieve the realisation of the one Tao or Brahman.

What this means in practical terms is that during love-making partners can allow themselves to manifest all the facets of their personalities and sexuality, thus achieving a level where they can experience unfeathered ecstasy. At this stage they taste again their limitless spiritual nature.

Ejaculatory Control

*E*JACULATORY CONTROL IS given great importance in the sexual practices of the East. There are two aspects of this discipline:

In the light of present day thinking, the first could be slightly controversial. Taoist and Tantric masters considered that the psychic and physical essence of man was concentrated in the semen and therefore by ejaculating men could lose their mental and bodily strength. Modern medicine does not consider seminal loss to be of such great importance; on the contrary within limits both male and female orgasms are seen as a means of relaxation and good health.

Some Taoist texts allow ejaculation as long as it is limited by age and health. In the books the *Secret Methods of the Plain Girl* and the *Sex Recipes of the Plain Girl*, where a Goddess instructs the mythical Yellow Emperor, it is stated:

> Every man should regulate the emission of semen according to his store of vital essence.
> He should never force himself to ejaculate.
> If he should do so, then his body will be harmed.
> A young and strong man can afford to ejaculate twice daily, but frail ones only once.
> A strong man of about thirty years of age can afford to do so once daily,
> whereas a weak man the same age should do so only every two days.
> A strong man of forty years can ejaculate once every three days,
> but a weak man this age should do so only every four days.

In modern terms, this means each man should become aware of the effects of ejaculation on his body. As long as it makes him feel happy and strong he should continue it, but when it starts to make him feel weak and lethargic he should limit it.

The second reason for controlling ejaculation is a sound one and can greatly enhance love-making.

Male sexuality centres on emission of semen and after orgasm the man tends to cease sexual activity, regardless of the woman's needs. If the man can control and delay orgasm he can prolong the sexual act allowing for exploration of various positions or simply for heightening and extending the pleasure of sensual caresses and physical contact. In this way love-making with all its facets – kissing, caressing, sensual massage and love positions – can be continued for hours if not for days. For certain Tantric practices it is advisable that the man maintains his erection without ejaculating, allowing him to move his penis inside the woman's vagina so that both partners have time to concentrate on the feelings generated by their physical union rather than just the quick sexual act. This is particularly important in Tantric Initiation.

The following is a useful and effective introductory exercise to help the man to delay or retain his orgasm.

Whilst making love the man should be careful not to overexcite himself to the point where he can no longer control his orgasm. If he feels himself climaxing he should slow down the rhythm of his strokes and gradually interrupt them. While leaving the penis in the vagina, he should relax his body and breathe slowly and deeply. His attention should be diverted from his genital sensations and focused instead on the pleasure of closeness and intimacy with his partner. He could, for example, exchange caresses, kisses or tender words. When he reassumes the penetrative strokes he should do so in a slow and relaxed way.

There is also a more advanced exercise for controlling ejaculation, which can be practised after the first exercise has been mastered.

When the man feels that he might be close to climaxing he should slow down or interrupt the strokes of his penis, whilst leaving his penis in the vagina, and he should take a deep and slow breath. During inspiration he should lightly contract the muscles between his anus and penis, together with his abdominal muscles. He should hold the contraction whilst he breathes in and out two or three times and then he should relax these muscles fully. After a few seconds he can repeat the cycle once or twice, then he can slowly reassume his love-making strokes.

With time the man will be able to control his ejaculation, prolonging at will the love-making session. After a rest lovers can restart their session, of course making sure that they are not unduly tiring themselves. They can repeat this pattern as long as they both wish.

Remember that the highest form of spirituality that these exercises can bring into your life is the happiness that you and your partner can give to each other. Love-making is just one way, probably the most enjoyable one, to touch that love – a love that knows no time.

Initiation

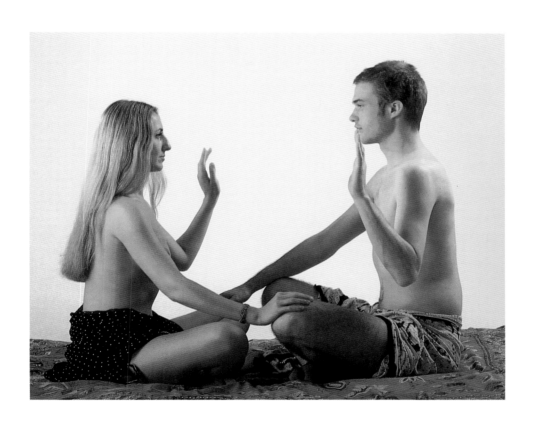

The Preparation

W HEN WRITING ABOUT Tantric and Taoist sexual and spiritual exercises the challenge one is faced with is that many of these rituals were reserved for the adept and keen student who was guided and monitored all the way by an advanced and experienced master. Tantric practices can open previously untapped psychic channels. This could, if it was not properly monitored, in some extreme cases cause a premature awakening of energies that the novice could not cope with. For this reason I have presented a series of simple meditative, sensual and sexual exercises and positions that are easy to follow and totally safe to practise. Despite their simplicity they will awaken new feelings of love and intimacy and prolong and heighten sexual joy.

The aim of the following initiatory or preparatory phase is to bring the partners closer together with loving feelings of tender care and with an awareness that by helping each other in their spiritual awakening they can not only vastly improve the quality of their relationship but also their overall quality of life. In this way relationships will not risk degenerating into boredom and apathy. On the contrary, they will remain fresh and a source of vigour and stimulation.

Eastern erotic and spiritual practices tell us never to rush things with a sense of anxiety and anticipation. On the contrary we should approach love-making and intimacy with calmness and with a sense of joyful timelessness. An emotional and physical contact coming from a caring heart is far more important than a rushed sexual session.

Before engaging in the various sexual positions and healing exercises the lovers should spend a few hours by themselves just pampering and cherishing each other. If they wished they could extend this session to a whole day or night.

Lovers should start by decorating their room in a warm and sensual way. They could try using sheets and covers made of such materials as satin or velvet in warm and voluptuous colours. Flowers and paintings could be used to embellish the room. If they feel adventurous and enthusiastic about the decoration they could also hang various draperies to create a sensation of being in a tent somewhere in the East.

The room should be warm but not stuffy and scented with oils, perfumes or incense. Lovers might like to take a bath together, or a shower. After this they could play some soft, pleasant and sensual music. Next they can either lie together softly talking and caressing each other or, even better, practising the sensual massage techniques. This alone could take a few hours. From time to time they could break for food and drink. I would advise colourful and warm items, for instance sensual fruits (such as strawberries, peaches or mangoes), heavily scented flowers (lilies, roses or freesias) and herbal teas (rosehip or hibiscus).

The couple should endeavour to bring delight and joy to one another by spending time caressing and massaging in favourite ways. It is a time for pampering each other and for confirming to one another that it is a real joy to be together.

During this time the couple should remain at a sensual and caring level of activity and should not engage in sexual contact. This is so they can later create a truly loving and sexual mood: remember that we are creating a totally new pathway of erotic communication.

CHILDREN

Many couples worry that it might not be easy for them to experience this sort of Tantric practice if they have children, particularly very young ones. In reality this is a very important time to practise sensual and caring exercises, as often children take up so much time and energy that the partners begin to lead separate lives and there is a need for them to come close again both emotionally and physically.

It is not essential to practise Tantra and Tao, particularly the above preparatory exercise, for a whole day. The occasional session for two to three hours while the children are asleep is sufficient to improve the love and pleasure in a couple's life.

This practice will not only benefit the couple and remove much of the stress which sometimes can crop up while raising children; but the joy in the parents will also reflect itself in a very positive way on the children.

Children should not be used as an excuse not to practise loving exercises. On the contrary, they should be a reason *to* practise them!

Not all of these exercises will be new to you – you have probably already explored some of them in your love-making. The emphasis of this book lies not only on the variety of positions that you can assume but on their capacity to generate a loving union and to heal physical, emotional and mental difficulties.

Tantric Initiation

WE HAVE ALREADY examined how Eastern thought views each part of creation as comprising both physical and mental attributes and therefore when massaging meridians or chakras we are not only soothing that particular body part but also initiating deeper psycho-physical changes. This is why during love-making while massaging areas of the body you are also improving the health of organs and releasing emotional blockages.

I again stress the fact that I have endeavoured to present the various healing exercises in an easy and simple way which is safe and effective for all to practise. If you are in doubt about your health you should consult your doctor before practising sexual healing exercises.

You will find that different ancient texts give different names to the same positions and sometimes this can be a bit disconcerting for the reader. Women have complained that some of the names are not very complimentary to them, for instance the Cow or the mounting of the Mare. Of course there is nothing wrong with animal names expressing love-making positions; the objection arises because of the connotation given by some people to those animal names. For this reason I have occasionally named a series of sexual positions by a general term and not worried unduly about the names of individual variations.

Remember that the exercises and massage techniques given in this book are not meant to be performed mechanically. The healing advice given will improve the erotic and sensual pleasure of the sexual act. The exercises aim to encourage you, during love-making, to use your hands, senses and imagination to give more pleasure and tenderness, and by soothing and opening your meridians and chakras to love in a deeper and more meaningful way.

The following exercises in particular express the true essence of Tantra and aim to show lovers how, even while keeping and strengthening their sense of personal identity, they can still create a sense of union and spiritual oneness. They can be practised purely as a meditation, or incorporated into love-making.

These exercises with their symbols and gestures aim to awaken in the couple their deepest love so that the sexual act will truly express the passion of their spirit. They can change for the better not only their relationship but also the general quality of their lives by reminding themselves that they will find true happiness only when they learn to relate to everyone in a loving and supportive way.

These exercises, if regularly practised for a few minutes each day or at least two or three times a week, can keep alight the candle of love and mutual respect that originally brought the couple together, and in most cases they can increase the power of this candle and give it new, exciting and long-lasting dimensions.

The exercises aim to show self-reliance to the couple so that they can love from a level of offering rather than need. They also remind both partners of the inherent beauty of their lover and that relationships should be based on mutual healing and genuine love.

As you practise these meditations you will notice that your relationship will increase in closeness, remove many of its obstacles and become a source of joy and healing.

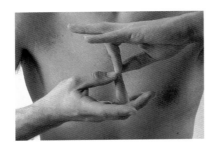

I am one with myself

This meditation is performed in order to awaken a feeling that we are not seeking a relationship in order to hide our solitude and lack of self love. Tantric love is born between two individuals who want to share and expand their inner beauty and creativity. Practise it for two to three minutes.

- Sit facing your partner in a meditative posture and practise the following Mudra (hand gesture).
- On each hand join the tips of your middle finger and thumb and keep your other three fingers straight.
- Join the tips of the middle fingers and thumbs of the two hands, the left hand on top and the right hand beneath and hold them in front of your stomach. This is a powerful symbol that signifies that the individual soul is united with the universal spirit unaffected by the changes of time (the thumb touching the middle finger). The joining of the left and right hands signifies that the female and male poles of the individual are in harmony.
- Now breathe slowly and deeply and inwardly feel that you are accomplished and contented as an individual and that your energies are in harmony. You should inwardly recite the following affirmation, 'I am complete within myself'.

I salute the divinity in you

Often when a relationship begins the partners see each other as an image of beauty and desire but as times goes by they start projecting a lot of negative images into each other. This meditation reminds them of the beautiful and divine nature of their partner and encourages them always to view the other in this light.

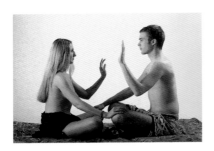

- Sit in front of your partner with your knees touching.
- Put your left hand on your partner's right knee and their right hand on your left knee.
- Raise your free hand so it is facing the heart or chest region of your partner.

- The man should first say, 'I salute the Goddess in you' to which the woman answers, 'I salute the God in you'. You can repeat the salutation two or three times.

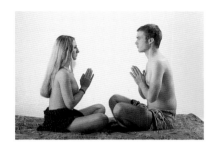

This pose can be used as a variation of the previous one.

- Sit facing your partner with your knees touching.
- Join your hands in the prayer position with the tips of your fingers slightly pointing towards the middle part of the chest of your partner.
- This position emphasises the heart-to-heart communication between the lovers.

Sharing the breath

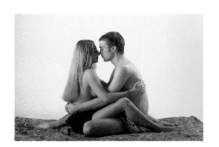

This breathing exercise reinforces the capacity to give and take unconditionally between the two lovers, bringing them closer to one another.

- Sit with your partner as shown in the illustration.
- Bring the tips of your noses close together.
- As you breathe out your partner should breathe in, inhaling your breath, and vice versa.
- Meditate on giving each other strength and support.
- This exercise should only be performed for about three minutes each time.

Understanding

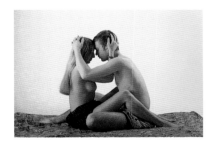

This exercise will bring your thoughts and perceptions even closer together, increasing your mental understanding, intuition and telepathy. You can practise it for about three to five minutes at a time twice a week.

- Sit as shown in the illustration and place your hands on each other's heads.
- Join your foreheads and concentrate on the area where your foreheads meet. Enjoy the warmth that this generates.

One breath

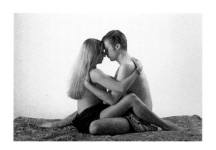

Now you are ready to experience a union of breaths and souls. This exercise will develop a sense of union and unconditional love recharging you both with vitality and healing power.

- Coordinate your breaths so that they follow the same rhythm of inhalation and exhalation.
- When you breathe in visualise a current of golden, warm energy rising along *the woman's* spine and reaching the top of your heads. When you breathe out visualise this healing energy descending along *the man's* spine, encircling the bottom of your pelvises and so on.
- You should feel that this energy is healing all your disharmonies at all levels, physical, mental and spiritual, making you both healthy and happy.
- You may like to repeat this exercise, changing the route of the visualisation, with the energy rising along *the man's* spine and descending down *the woman's* spine.

Healing light

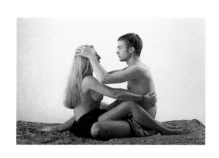

This is a powerful exercise to bring healing and happiness into your life, reminding you that your bond should be formed by true love and a sincere desire for the happiness of your partner.

- Raise your hands in the air as shown on page 26 and visualise that you are receiving a golden, loving and healing light in the palms of your hands.
- After a minute or so turn your palms down and place them over the head of your partner. Feel the light entering him or her from the head to the toes, filling him or her with joy and healing
- Truly wish your partner happiness and well-being. The exercise can last for about three to five minutes.
- Next your partner can repeat the exercise on you, to bring you healing.

Creating power

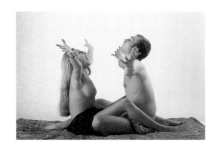

Much too often when we cannot achieve our aims in life due to our own incapacity we become frustrated and tend to vent anger on our partner. In this way we can greatly undermine the relationship. Anger and blame make us weak and destroy love. This exercise aims to release anger and frustration, transforming them into a source of power.

- Raise your arms wide apart and open your mouths and jaws as far as you can.
- Emit roaring sounds of anger trying to resemble the roaring of a tiger.
- When you feel a small amount of vibration rippling through your bodies, the exercise is achieving its aim to liberate blocked and frustrated energies.
- Practise for two minutes twice a week if needed.

The warm embrace

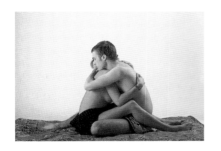

If practised for a few minutes each time, this exercise will instill into the relationship a quality of timeless love and togetherness.

- Hold each other as shown in the illustration. The embrace should be quite tight but in no way should it feel uncomfortable or unpleasant. The aim is to convey a feeling of unity and caring.
- Visualise and feel that you are both becoming one light and one body and that your love knows no boundaries.

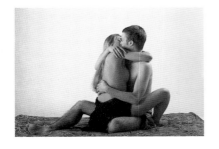

From the previous exercise, *The Warm Embrace*, you can go straight into a passionate kiss. It is a beautiful and poetical way to finish this section and it also seals the effects of the other exercises with one of the most tender expressions of love.

Sexual positions:
man on top

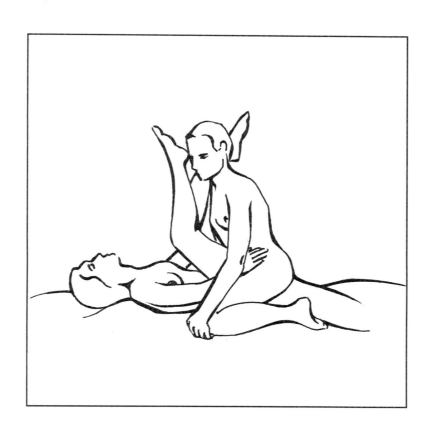

*T*HERE IS A SYMBOLISM associated both with the man on top and woman on top positions. As I described in earlier chapters, although man and woman have physical attributes that link the first to the Yang or dynamic force and the latter to the Yin or receptive force, in reality neither of them is fully Yang or Yin. Both man and woman contain Yin and Yang qualities within themselves, in the same way that men carry female hormones and women carry male hormones.

Tantra, in particular, strongly emphasises this point and for this reason it often portrays women on top of men and Goddesses on top of Gods. The important thing to remember is that, regardless of who is on top, both partners should offer their deepest love and healing potential.

When the man is on top he should meditate on himself as the carrier of the vital seed (sperm). He should visualise himself as a tall, strong tree germinating and laying seeds over the earth. He should feel proud of his strength and grateful to the earth for its receptivity. The seeds he carries on a mental level represent countless life forms and the infinite possibilities of a creative and active mind.

To spread one's seed onto the earth means to be active, alive and participating at all times with the process of existence. It means to infuse spirit and initiative into all of our actions and endeavours.

What this also symbolises is that to be truly sexual one needs to be a dynamic, resourceful and creative person. It also means that a spirited person will have more energy to offer to his or her love-making and that happy love-making can also make a person more dynamic and spirited.

The woman in these positions where she is more receptive, although in these love-making techniques she is also participating with her healing caresses, can meditate on the power of receptiveness. She should feel happy to receive the dynamic power of the Yang force and know that by letting herself be receptive she acquires the joy and power of the whole earth.

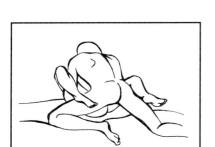

The missionary position

This section begins with the most known and practised position, which is known in the West as the Missionary pose. It is the position that is found most natural during intercourse and that over the centuries people have sometimes adhered to monotonously, either because of lack of imagination or because of a sense of prudishness and shame. However, it is a comfortable and easy position and I shall show you how to use it as a starting position from which you can flow into a wide variety healing and erotic embraces. In ancient Eastern texts it is often referred to as the Opening Flower, a definition I like because it denotes an erotic beginning and an opening to love.

Healing effect

Establishes a sense of security and trust in both partners which they can build on later on when they come to explore different positions.

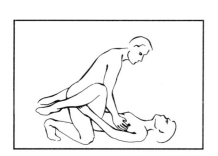

A variation on the missionary position

- Hold your body slightly more upright than in the missionary position
- With your hands caress your partner's breasts and shoulders using a circular motion. Start with your hands together positioned over the tip of her breast bone, pointing towards her head.
- Glide your hands over your partner's chest until they reach the top.
- Next continue the gliding movement encircling her shoulders and following the outer contours of her breasts until you return to the original position.
- Continue this until you both find it pleasurable.

Healing effect

This stroke improves digestion, strengthens the lungs and heart and creates a very pleasant sensation across the torso.

Variation 2: Releasing the neck

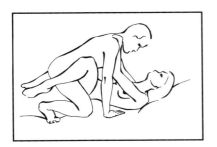

- In this variation, extend your legs so that you can rest comfortably on your hands and closer to your partner.
- She can now massage the muscles of your shoulders in a sensual and deep manner.

Healing effect

In this way your partner can release in you deeply stored tension that often accumulates in the shoulder area, thus allowing you to feel even more relaxed during love-making. This technique is also useful to relieve tension headaches in the man.

Variation 3: Raising the pelvis

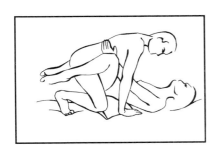

- In this position place a cushion beneath the buttocks of your partner. In this way you raise her pelvis allowing for deeper penetration and intimacy.
- As in all positions that allow deeper penetration you should be careful not to hurt your partner and should perform your love strokes in a gentle and sensitive way.

Healing effect

This position creates feelings of warmth and intimacy. It helps to release tension and to improve the functioning of the kidneys.

Variation 4: Caressing the upper leg

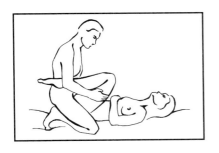

This is a good position for you to massage the upper part of your partner's legs.

- Place both hands on top of your partner's knees with fingertips facing each other.
- Next glide your hands along the outer margin of her thighs until they reach the pelvic area.

◆ Return to the original position by massaging the inner part of the upper thigh.

Healing effect

This massage movement releases tension in the upper legs encouraging trust and enjoyment.

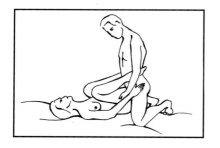

The Indrani

In India this position is called *Indrani* because it was said that it was greatly enjoyed by the wife of the god Indra. All the techniques in this section can shorten the woman's vagina and allow for deeper penetration, and although this can greatly increase intimacy and heighten sexual pleasure, be careful not to thrust too hard and hurt her. You should also be sensitive to her pelvic movements and directions.

These positions allow for a love-making technique where the penis moves in a circular motion inside the vagina rather than in straight thrusts, a penetrative variation that is greatly enjoyed by many women.

Healing effect

The Indrani releases nervous tension, particularly in the woman.

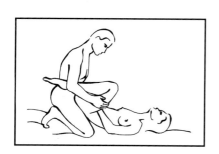

A variation on the Indrani

In this variation of Indrani you can massage the whole length of the outer part of your partner's leg.

◆ Place one hand with your fingers pointing upwards on the outer side of your partner's ankle and massage the whole length of her leg up to the border of the thigh.

◆ Return to the original position and continue if you both find it pleasurable.

Healing effect

This massage stroke is helpful to reduce accumulation of fluids and cellulite in the leg. It also improves the gall-bladder meridian, thereby improving digestion. By treating the gall-bladder meridian you can also release frustration and anger.

Sweet Love

When the woman places her feet over the man's chest the position is called *Sweet Love*. This position allows deeper penetration.

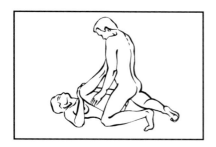

- ◆ Your partner lies on her back with her legs raised and bent at the knee.
- ◆ She rests her feet on your chest, while you move inside her.

Healing effect

The woman is able to stimulate the man's heart chakra with her feet, increasing his feelings of love.

A variation on Sweet Love

This variation of Sweet Love is similar to the one of Indrani but it does offer a different angle of penetration and massage.

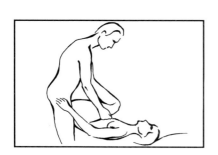

- ◆ Place both hands above your partner's ankles with your fingertips facing one another.
- ◆ Massage the top of her thighs by gliding your palms all the way up to the pelvic border.
- ◆ Return to her ankles, gliding your hands along the outer part of her legs.

Healing effect

In this way you massage the stomach, and gall-bladder meridians, improving digestion and helping with the elimination of accumulation of fluids and cellulite.

By massaging these meridians you also help your partner to release anger and frustration and at the same time acquire a sense of grounding and tranquillity.

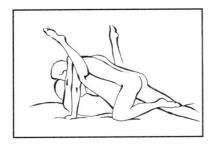

The Yawning position

This pose is called the *Yawning* position. It stretches and tightens the muscles of the woman's legs and allows for greater movement.

- Ask your partner to raise her legs as far as she can do so comfortably. She might like to rest her legs against your sides.
- Lean forward slightly to enable you to penetrate her more deeply.

Healing effect

Strengthens the man's kidneys and adrenals, and the woman's legs. It also stimulates lymphatic drainage in the woman, thus helping to eliminate cellulite.

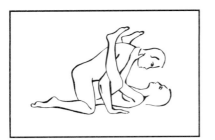

A variation of Yawning

- You can help keep your partner's legs in this position by gently pressing down against her thighs with your arms. This allows for further dilation of her vagina and deeper penetration.
- Your partner is in a good position to gently squeeze and massage your neck muscles giving you a very sensual and pleasant sensation of relaxation.

Healing effect

This position is relaxing for both partners and releases tension in the man. It allows for a greater sense of intimacy and penetrative pleasure.

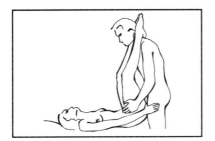

Caressing raised legs

- In this position your partner rests her legs on your shoulders with her feet close to your neck.
- Massage her leg in the same way as in the Sweet Love variation.

Healing effect

This position offers your partner a comfortable way to stretch and strengthen her leg muscles.

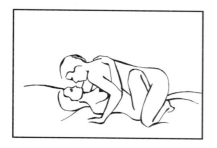

The Lotus

This a very poetical and symbolical position called the *Lotus*.

- Your partner should rest her left foot on her right thigh and pull her right foot up her left leg as far as is comfortable.
- The lotus flower represents love and spiritual perfection. Your partner should feel that she is a happy spiritual being whilst you should feel grateful and joyful to be making love to her.

Healing effect

This position enhances the spiritual love each partner feels, transforming the union of bodies into the union of souls.

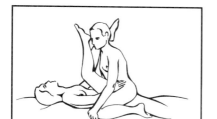

Raising and lowering the legs

- While having her legs upright against your shoulders, your partner should raise then lower her legs slowly.
- This movement creates a sense of very pleasant and varied sensations caused by her vagina relaxing and tightening.

Healing effect

This position not only increases the pleasure, but can also strengthen your partner's legs.

Sexual positions:
woman on top

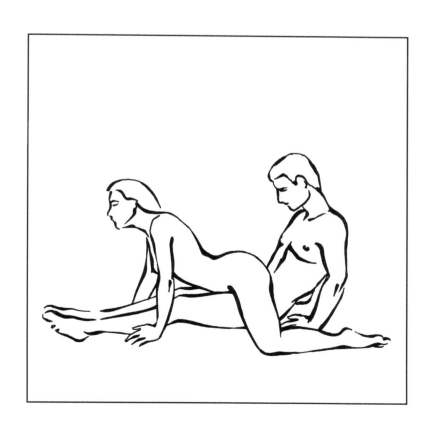

*A*s MENTIONED IN THE chapter Man on Top, woman is also Yang and man is also Yin and Tantra strongly emphasises this point by repeatedly portraying the symbol of the Goddess as the power of the universe sitting or dancing on top of a God.

Tantra and also Taoism teach that although most traditional societies tried to portray women almost exclusively as a receptive and compliant figure and the Yin symbol as a symbol of submissive passivity, the female principle is in reality the more active and creative force in the universe.

The female body with its roundness and fecundity strongly represents the qualities of the earth but when the woman comes in touch with her deeper essence she turns into fire and wind – the dynamic aspects of the elements.

The man becomes passive but in the process achieves peace and tranquillity because he drops all the pretences of perennial strength and false power. By surrendering to the power of the Goddess and renouncing his continuous sense of strife and struggle, he achieves a new sense of peace and inner joy.

The woman enters in touch with her inner power and sees herself as the force of creation firing up all the universe and giving life to all forms. She is filled with force and compassion, and is endowed with a power which is also filled with love.

These positions not only aim to procure enhanced sexual pleasure, they also encourage the couple to view sexual and gender roles in a changeable and dynamic way which can only benefit both partners, particularly the woman.

These positions reverse the traditional notion of the male being the active and dominating partner and they give the woman the capacity to express her sexuality, power and healing abilities. In Tantra the female pole, also called *Shakti*, is in reality the creative and dynamic force that animates all of creation, which is why many Tantric texts give great importance to these positions.

Woman on top

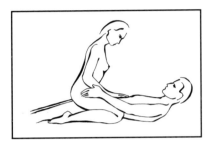

In this position the woman can express her power and sexuality, reversing the traditional role of her being the more passive partner. Tantra views the female force as the creative power of the universe and these positions allow her to manifest this force.

- Sit astride your partner, bending your legs at the knee.
- Once you are comfortably in position, draw your partner's penis deep within you.

Healing Effect

This position increases the energy flow in your body, as well as creating a sense of freedom.

Opening the chest

- Start with your hands together positioned over the tip of your partner's breast bone, pointing towards his head.
- Glide your hands together until they reach the top of his chest.
- Continue the gliding movement encircling his shoulders and following the outer contours of his chest until you are back at the original position.
- Continue if you both find it pleasurable.

Healing Effect

This is a very pleasurable stroke that can also improve the health of the respiratory system and soothe the heart.

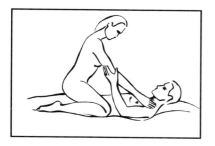

Caressing the arms

- Your partner places both palms, with his fingers pointing upwards, on your wrists and glides them up your arms with a soft massage stroke all the way to the shoulders.
- Then he turns his fingers downwards and with a circular movement returns with the same gliding motion to your wrists.
- He repeats this stroke in a steady rhythm if you both so wish.

Healing Effect

This stroke massages various meridians including the large intestine and small intestine, helping digestion and soothing abdominal spasms.

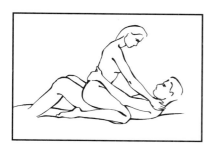

Drawing closer

- Your partner slightly raises his legs to help you to lean forwards.
- Place your hands over his neck, massaging it in a slow and sensual way.

Healing Effect

This technique soothes neck stiffness, helping conditions such as tension headaches, as well as relaxing the male into the pleasures of love-making.

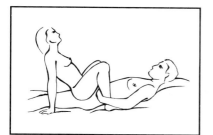

Expressing power

- Lean backwards arching your shoulders and opening your chest.
- You then can increase the rhythm of your strokes.
- Emit any sounds that you deem fit to express your feelings at the moment.

Healing Effect

This technique encourages the woman to manifest her anger and express her power and individuality.

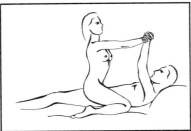

The Grip

- Both you and your partner should interlace your fingers in a firm but not painful or uncomfortable grip.
- Concentrate on the strength of your grip and on the power that your love-making is generating.

Healing Effect

This position enables each partner to transmit energy and strength to the other, and increase stamina.

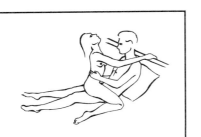

The Anchor

This variation can be more comfortable for some men allowing them more participation. It also allows the woman to anchor herself more firmly over the man achieving a deeper penetration.

- Your partner sits with his back resting against the headboard of a bed or similar.
- Sit astride your partner, with your knees slightly raised. Stabilise yourself by holding the headboard, if necessary.
- While you move, gently arch your back and tilt your head back.

Healing effect

This position raises energy and stimulates the imaginative and creative faculties of the couple.

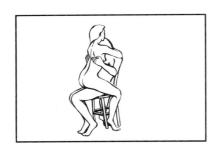

The Chair

This position again can be highly erotic allowing a deeper embrace and penetration between the lovers and dispensing also with the need for a bed, allowing love-making anywhere there is a chair!

- Your partner sits on a high back chair, feet firmly planted on the ground, keeping his back straight.
- Sit astride your partner. Place your arms around his back while he holds you close.

Healing effect

This position generates a feeling of intimacy and releases each partner's creative energy as it stimulates the chakras located in the abdomen. It also improves digestion.

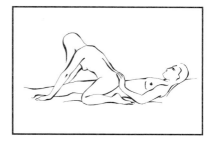

The Reversed Role

This is an erotic variation that gives the man a beautiful view of his partner's body.

- Sit astride your partner, with your back to him.
- You could also caress and massage the top part of your partner's legs.

Healing effect

Massaging your partner's legs stimulates his energy flow, the lymphatic system and circulation. You are very likely to experience a sense of release.

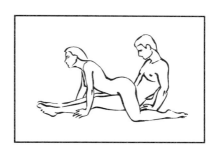

A variation on the Reversed Role

- Sit astride your partner with your back to him, then lean forwards over his legs with your head over his feet.
- This position allows you to experiment with pelvic movements.

Healing effect

This position strengthens your arms and legs. It also increases stamina.

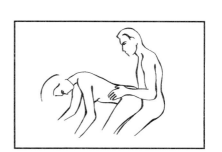

A second variation on the Reversed Role

As I mentioned earlier there is something very erotic about making love over a chair, particularly because it dispenses with the need for a bed and allows the passion of love-making to flow in most places!

- Your partner sits in a high back chair, with his back straight.
- With your back to your partner and leaning slightly forward, sit on his lap.
- He will then be able to massage and scratch your lower back gently, while you move against him.

Healing effect

This position enables your partner to facilitate the energy flow from your lower back to the rest of your body.

Sexual positions: other ideas

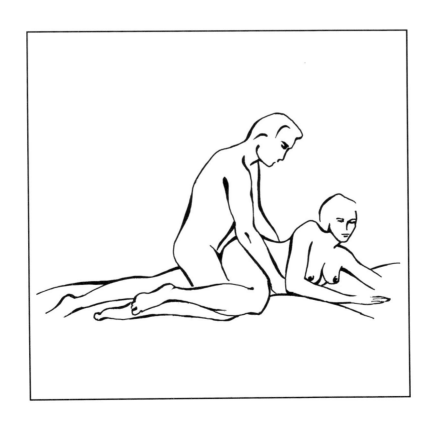

Man behind the woman

THIS IS A WAY of making love that can be quite instinctual and a derivation of our animal past as most animals copulate in this way. It allows deeper penetration and stimulation of the G spot in the woman. The penis can also, with a variety of movements, reach and stimulate many parts of the vagina that otherwise it could not have reached. Again thanks to the Tantric and Taoist understanding of energy these positions can also be used for healing and improving stamina.

Resting together

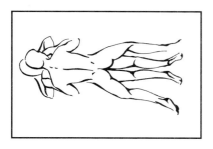

- Your partner should lie comfortably on her stomach with her arms by her sides. It is advisable to put a cushion or pillow under her pelvis; this lifts her buttocks making penetration easier and more pleasurable for both.
- After penetration gently rest on her, with your head on her upper back and your arms encircling her shoulders. You should both enjoy the proximity and warmth of your contact.

Healing effect

This position allows deeper penetration, while creating a sense of relaxation and trust between the partners.

Raising the energy

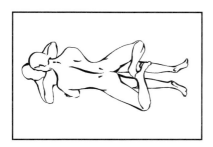

- Lie your partner comfortably on her stomach with her head resting on her folded arms.
- Place your hands on the floor and rest your weight on your arms.
- Slightly arch your back.
- Breathe deeply and slowly and concentrate on your back area at the level of the waist where your kidneys and adrenal glands are located.

Healing effect

Taoism believes that this is a vital area for generating energy and the man should visualise that his kidney area is generating a lot of vitality with making love in this position. The woman can concentrate as well on the warmth and energy that she is feeling in the lower back area.

Creating a sense of warmth and intimacy

This is a lovely variation of the two previous techniques creating a great sense of warmth and intimacy.

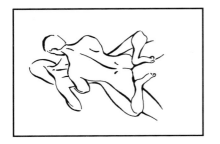

- With your partner still lying face down, you should encircle her body with your arms.
- She will then bring her feet up towards your buttocks, allowing deeper penetration.

Healing effect

This position encourages trust and communication. The more couples communicate, the more happiness and pleasure they will experience.

A variation with woman raising her body

This is probably one of the most popular positions practised by individuals who view sex with a more liberal mind. The position is sometimes unkindly referred to as the 'cow' in the East or as 'doggy' in the West, not that the visions of animals making love is not poetic but in some people these words trigger less poetical images.

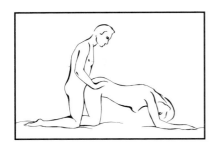

- Gently raise your partner's buttocks until she is supporting her weight on her knees and hands.
- Hold your partner's waist to allow deeper penetration and to give you greater stability.

Healing effect

This position affords deep but gentle penetration and gives a very good angle for the man to stimulate the G spot in the woman's vagina.

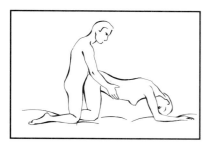

Variation 2: Caressing the sides of the body

- Place both hands together with your palms down and fingers pointing upwards at the base of your partner's spine.
- Massage her back by gliding both hands together covering both sides of the spine.
- When you reach the top turn your fingers outwards and encircle her shoulders, rubbing them.
- Return to the original position, massaging her sides as you go.
- Continue this effleurage in a steady rhythm as long as you both enjoy it.

Healing effect

Massaging the back in this fashion is very soothing and regulates the many nerves that emerge from the spine, thus improving the whole body.

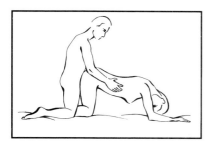

Variation 3: Closer together

- Stroke your partner in a similar way to the previous technique but this time concentrate your massage on her lower back and buttocks.

Healing effect

This stroke can improve the functioning of the kidneys and reproductive system.

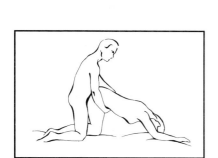

Variation 4: Drawing closer

- Ask your partner to bend forwards and down lowering her arms and raising her pelvis closer to you.
- From this position you can reach her clitoris more easily and gently stimulate it.
- This position brings your pelvises very close together and gives your partner both external and internal stimulation.

Healing effect

This position stretches your partner's back, improving the flow of energy up the spine. The revitalising effects of this can be felt throughout the body.

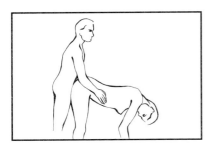

Variation 5: Woman standing

This is a position that can be practised easily almost anywhere in the house.

◆ While you are both standing, ask your partner to lean over a stool or chair.

Healing effect

As with the previous position, this variant improves the energy flow up the spine and revitalises the whole body.

Closer Together

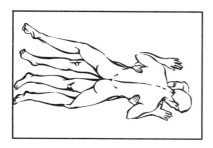

$\mathcal{T}$HIS INTIMATE POSITION is often referred to as the Box, representing the closeness between the two lovers. In this way the woman can exert a powerful grip on the penis with the muscles of her vagina.

- With your partner lying on her back, gently lower yourself on top of her, with your legs slightly parted.
- You can hold her head tenderly in your hands, while she embraces you.

Healing effect

The lovers should meditate on the warmth generated in their heart region in the chest and see it as an expression of their timeless love.

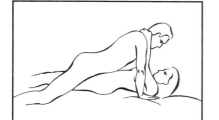

A variation on the Box

- Following on from the previous position, extend your back, leaning on your arms and continue your love-making in this position.
- Your partner can raise her arms and massage your neck with deep and warm strokes.

Healing effect

This stroke releases tension in the neck and relieves head-aches.

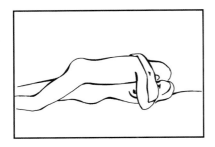

Variation 2: Closer together

This position can bring you as lovers closer than ever to one another. You should feel your hearts and bodies melting together.

◆ Embrace your partner warmly, while she draws you tightly to her.

Healing effect

As for the previous variants, this position creates a sense of intimacy.

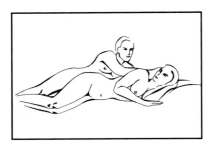

Gentle Love

◆ Lie behind your partner.
◆ Slightly turn her pelvis and flex her legs so that you can penetrate her.
◆ Make love to her slowly and gently whilst caressing her hair, head and body with a sense of warmth and care.
◆ You should both enjoy the languor, relaxation and timelessness of the moment.

Healing effect

This position creates a sense of relaxation and langour, removing the constraints of time and routine.

Splitting of a Bamboo

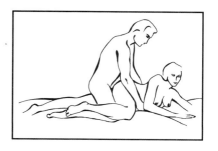

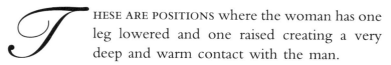HESE ARE POSITIONS where the woman has one leg lowered and one raised creating a very deep and warm contact with the man.

- Ask your partner to lie on her side with her left leg straight and her right leg bent.
- Kneel with one knee on each side of the straight leg. This position tightens the vaginal walls giving the penetration a major sense of fullness.

Healing effect

This is quite a pictorial position! As you can see in sex there are no limits for those with imagination and a sense of fun.

A variation on Splitting of a Bamboo

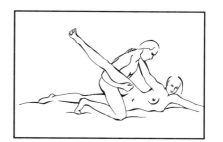

- Using the same basic position, take your partner's right leg and hold it straight over your leg.
- Your partner can then caress your neck.

Healing effect

This position stimulates the imagination and encourages playfulness.

Variation 2: Resting leg on man's shoulder

This position is for the woman who is athletically minded, and who has flexible limbs.

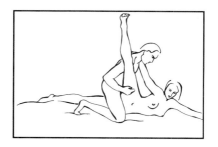

- Still in the same position, now your partner could bend her leg and rest it against your neck.

Healing effect

This position can greatly strengthen and tone your partner's leg muscles.

Conclusion

♦   ♦   ♦   ♦   ♦

*B*ROWSING THROUGH ANY bookshop we can see that there many books on sexuality, most of which have a useful role to play and some positive advice to offer. Some deal mainly with sexual problems of a physical nature, some aim to help us to remove emotional blockages that hamper a happy sexual relationship, while others describe a great variety of sexual poses and techniques.

This book can help relationships at different levels as it includes aspects of human sexuality, but above all it aims to help people build a happier relationship based on a love that includes a spiritual as well as a physical dimension. It fulfils this task by drawing inspiration from the ancient Eastern paths.

Traditional thought in the West has had a tendency to view sex purely as an act of procreation, of which we should almost be ashamed and embarrassed. Modern society has tried to counteract this narrow view by creating one that presents sex as an act of mere pleasure and release.

The time has come to unite sexuality with spirituality. I use the word spirituality in a very simple and down-to-earth manner, not as some sort of mysterious and esoteric expression. To me to be spiritual means to love from the depths of one's heart, to mean it and to show it through one's actions, and there is no better place to start than in one's own home.

Tantra is a great stepping stone on the way to achieve this aim because it shows a way to be loving and caring while at the same time having a good time and enjoying oneself.

Sex *is* an act of procreation but it does not necessarily have to lead to offspring. It is a way of celebrating life and the joy of relationships. According to Tantra and Taoism, sex is an act of worship which tremendously improves our lives at many levels.

Sexual Healing improves communication when people have ceased talking and relating, it reminds us of the love in our hearts when we tend to forget it, it makes us better human beings when we tend to become resentful and aloof, and above all it keeps the flame of passion and sexual joy alight when it starts becoming feeble.

I wish you all many happy hours, days and years filled with passion and peace and may your inner happiness shine to all the world!